W9-BXW-069

STUDENT WORKBOOK

Administrative Medical Assisting

Foundations and Practices, 2e

CHRISTINE MALONE
MBA, MHA, CMPE, CPHRM, FACHE

PEARSON

Publisher: Julie Levin Alexander
Publisher's Assistant: Regina Bruno
Acquisitions Editor: Marlene Pratt
Program Manager: Faye Gemmellaro
Editorial Assistant: Lauren Bonilla
Development Editor: Alexis Ferraro, iD8-TripleSSS Media
    Development, LLC
Marketing Manager: Brittany Hammond
Senior Marketing Coordinator: Alicia Wozniak
Marketing Specialist: Michael Sirinides
Project Management, Team Lead: Cindy Zonneveld
Project Manager: Yagnesh Jani
Full-Service Project Management: Kailash Jadli/
    Aptara®, Inc.
Senior Operations Specialist: Mary Ann Gloriande
Digital Program Manager: Amy Peltier
Media Project Manager: Lorena Cerisano
Creative Director: Andrea Nix
Art Director: Maria Guglielmo Walsh
Cover and Interior Designer: Ilze Lemesis
Cover Image: manaemedia/shutterstock
Composition: Aptara®, Inc.

Notice: The authors and the publisher of this volume have taken care that the information and technical recommendations contained herein are based on research and expert consultation and are accurate and compatible with the standards generally accepted at the time of publication. Nevertheless, as new information becomes available, changes in clinical and technical practices become necessary. The reader is advised to carefully consult manufacturers' instructions and information material for all supplies and equipment before use, and to consult with a health care professional as necessary. This advice is especially important when using new supplies or equipment for clinical purposes. The authors and publisher disclaim all responsibility for any liability, loss, injury, or damage incurred as a consequence, directly or indirectly, of the use and application of any of the contents of this volume.

Copyright © 2015, 2010 by Pearson Education, Inc. or its affiliates. All Rights Reserved. Printed in the United States of America. This publication is protected by copyright, and permission should be obtained from the publisher prior to any prohibited reproduction, storage in a retrieval system, or transmission in any form or by any means, electronic, mechanical, photocopying, recording, or otherwise. For information regarding permissions, request forms and the appropriate contacts within the Pearson Education Global Rights & Permissions department, please visit www.pearsoned.com/permissions/

Many of the designations by manufacturers and seller to distinguish their products are claimed as trademarks. Where those designations appear in this book, and the publisher was aware of a trademark claim, the designations have been printed in initial caps or all caps.

PEARSON

ISBN-13: 978-0-13-343074-5
ISBN-10:   0-13-343074-X

Contents

INTRODUCTION

This student workbook is designed to accompany *Administrative Medical Assisting: Foundations and Practices, 2e* as a study guide and practice tool. Complete each exercise in the chapters of this workbook as they correspond with the chapters of your student textbook to help reinforce and supplement what you have already learned.

Each chapter of this student workbook includes the following:

Chapter Outline: This is an outline of the topics that were covered in the corresponding chapter of your student textbook. If any of the content of the outline is unfamiliar, it is recommended that you go back to the book and look over that section.

Chapter Review: This is a summary of the main topics presented in the chapter.

Learning Activities: These questions and activities assess whether or not you have learned and retained the information presented in the text.

Applied Learning Exercises: These additional questions and activities further test your knowledge of the material presented in the chapter and may require additional research on the Internet or through another source.

Terminology Review: Key terms from the chapter are presented in the terminology review section of each chapter. You will be asked to write the definition of each key term. Abbreviations from the student text are also presented, and you will be asked to write the meaning of each.

Critical Thinking Questions: These critical thinking questions are built around real-life scenarios and provide you the opportunity to test your knowledge of key concepts presented in the chapter.

Chapter Review Test: The chapter review test consists of multiple choice, true/false, and short answer questions and is provided for additional practice and assessment.

An appendix of competency skill check-off sheets appears at the end of this workbook.

Answers to questions in this workbook can be found in the Instructor's Resource Manual.

CHAPTER 1

The History of Medicine and Health Care

CHAPTER OUTLINE

CHAPTER REVIEW

- Medicine has been practiced for many centuries with each culture practicing its own methods to treat and cure the ailments common at the time. Many of the health care practices seen in traditional Western medicine today have their roots in the ancient medical practices of long ago.

- The profession of medical assisting has seen many advances since its introduction to the medical professions. As the scope of practice for medical assistants expands, so will the need for continuing education in the field.

- Over the last 200 or so years, health care advances have made great strides, resulting in the discovery of X-rays, medications, and anesthesia. These three areas alone have dramatically transformed how society thinks about disease.

- Many of today's vaccinations were discovered in the 20th century, as were nearly all currently prescribed medications. The development of these vaccinations led to the treatment and prevention of diseases such as polio and chickenpox.

- The discovery of DNA in the 1950s paved the way for scientists in the 1990s to launch the Human Genome Project, an initiative aimed at identifying all the genes in human DNA. The research from this project has been used by scientists to determine if people have predispositions to such conditions as cancer, blood-clotting disorders, cystic fibrosis, and liver disease.

- Scientists believe that the biggest advances in medicine will be in the area of prevention of disease.

- Physicians today have ready access to numerous electronic resources where health care information can be accessed immediately.

© 2015 Pearson Education, Inc.

- A number of longstanding, pivotal organizations have formed throughout the years to further the advances of medical knowledge and achievement. These include, but are not limited to, the American Hospital Association (AHA), the American Medical Association (AMA), and the World Health Organization (WHO).

- Women, including Clara Barton, Marie Curie, Florence Nightingale, Elizabeth Blackwell, and Emily Blackwell, have played a significant role in medicine throughout modern history.

- Health care will likely continue to yield critical discoveries. Among the promising areas of research are stem cell research, transplants, and chemistry in the area of pharmacology.

- The Patient Protection and Affordable Care Act, also known as Obamacare, was signed into law in March 2010. This law mandates a system that provides and offers health care coverage for all Americans.

- Today, the use of evidence-based medicine is common practice. This philosophy is built on the premise that health care treatments should be based on scientific findings, randomized controlled trials, and medical literature to find the most effective ways to treat disease.

- Traditionally, physicians hired nurses to work in their offices. With a shortage of nurses, physicians began to seek other qualified staff that could fulfill administrative and clinical duties. As a result, the demand for formally trained medical assistants began to rise. Today, medical assistants of both sexes are well-trained, valuable members of the health care team.

LEARNING ACTIVITIES

To ensure that you have achieved the learning objectives in this chapter:

1. In the Terminology Review section on page 3, define the key terminology found in this chapter of your student text.

2. Create a list of the significant medical advances that have occurred throughout history. Next to each one, describe how that medical advancement is still used today or has paved the way for treatments or therapies that are used today.

_____

_____

_____

_____

_____

_____

APPLIED LEARNING EXERCISES

Using a separate sheet of paper, complete the following assignments:

1. Using the Internet, research some aspect relating to the history of medicine and health care that is not covered in this chapter. Write a 1–2-page essay describing your findings.

2. Choose one of the early medical practices of the cultures/societies mentioned in this chapter. Using the Internet or other research source, write a 1–2-page essay describing your findings.

3. Choose one of the health care pioneers discussed in this chapter. Using the Internet or other research source, write a 1–2-page essay describing the contributions this person made to the field of health care.

© 2015 Pearson Education, Inc.

TERMINOLOGY REVIEW

Using the glossary and highlighted terms in the textbook, define the following terms:

American Association of Medical Assistants (AAMA): _____

_____

American Red Cross: _____

_____

anatomy: _____

_____

anesthesia: _____

_____

antisepsis: _____

_____

astrology: _____

_____

autopsy: _____

_____

caduceus: _____

_____

chiropractic: _____

_____

chloroform: _____

_____

ether: _____

_____

evidence-based medicine: _____

_____

faith healer: _____

_____

Hippocrates: _____

_____

Human Genome Project: _____

_____

pharmaceuticals: _____

_____

physiology: _____

_____

public health: _____

_____

radiocarbon dating: _____

shaman: _____

ultrasound: _____

ABBREVIATIONS

Provide the meanings of the following abbreviations:

AAMA: _____

AHA: _____

AMA: _____

CT: _____

DNA: _____

ECG: _____

FAA: _____

JAMA: _____

MRI: _____

TB: _____

WHO: _____

CRITICAL THINKING QUESTIONS

1. Michelle Manwiller, CMA (AAMA), is working with Harold Chan, a 55-year-old patient. Mr. Chan tells Michelle that he would like to try Chinese medicine treatments instead of taking the medication the physician has prescribed. He asks Michelle if she is familiar with the philosophy behind Chinese medicine. How might Michelle answer?

   _____

   _____

   _____

   _____

   _____

2. Robert Bautista is taking an administrative medical assisting course as part of his training to earn a certificate in medical assisting. He has been asked to write a paragraph outlining the contributions the Greek physician Galen made to medicine. Robert has been told to include the reasons why Galen's findings were not completely accurate. What could Robert write on this topic?

   _____

   _____

© 2015 Pearson Education, Inc.

_____

_____

_____

_____

3. Willie Harrison, a medical assisting student, has been assigned to write a brief essay on the history of the use of anesthesia in medicine. What important dates and information should Willie include in his timeline of the history of anesthesia?

_____

_____

_____

_____

_____

_____

4. Kristine Alberto, RMA (AMT), is working with Elizabeth Rashenko, a six-month-old patient. The physician has ordered a series of vaccines for Elizabeth, and Elizabeth's mother questions Kristine about the vaccines. Elizabeth's mother wants to know how long vaccines have been used in this country. The vaccines include influenza, polio (oral), measles, mumps, rubella, and chicken pox. How might Kristine answer this mother's question?

_____

_____

_____

_____

_____

_____

5. Marian Reiman, CMA (AAMA), is teaching a night class to medical assisting students. Marian wants to lecture on the different types of hospitals that currently exist in the United States. What are the four categories of hospitals she should talk about, and how should she describe one of these categories?

_____

_____

_____

_____

_____

_____

CHAPTER REVIEW TEST

MULTIPLE CHOICE

Circle the letter of the correct answer.

1. Early European medicine used _____ to train physicians.
   a. astrology
   b. cadavers
   c. animals
   d. live patients
   e. None of the above

2. In early Native American medicine, _____ was considered one of the highest forms of bravery.
   a. becoming a medicine man
   b. using Chinese medicine techniques
   c. suicide
   d. euthanizing sick patients
   e. performing surgery

3. Imhotep is credited as founding _____ medicine in the Third Dynasty.
   a. Roman
   b. Chinese
   c. Japanese
   d. Egyptian
   e. English

4. Cave paintings discovered in the _____ caves in France depict people using plants and herbs to treat illness.
   a. Caduceus
   b. Shaman
   c. Lascaux
   d. Rousseau
   e. Algerian

5. _____ is known as the "Father of Medicine."
   a. Galen
   b. Lister
   c. Vesalius
   d. Hippocrates
   e. Jenner

6. Surgeon _____, who lived from 1728 to 1793, developed many of the surgical techniques that are still used today.
   a. Jenner
   b. Hunter
   c. Laënnec
   d. Galen
   e. Curie

7. American physician and pharmacist _____ was the first to use modern anesthesia, in 1842.
   a. Galen
   b. Jenner
   c. Long
   d. Lister
   e. Curie

© 2015 Pearson Education, Inc.

8. _____ discovered X-rays in 1895.
   a. Roentgen
   b. Semmelweiss
   c. Galen
   d. Vesalius
   e. Jenner

9. Which of the following vaccines was developed prior to 1950?
   a. Chicken pox
   b. Pertussis
   c. Rubella
   d. Oral polio
   e. Shingles

10. The American Medical Association was founded in what year?
   a. 1800
   b. 1825
   c. 1847
   d. 1902
   e. 2004

TRUE/FALSE

Identify whether the statement is true (T) or false (F).

_____ 1. The Red Cross was founded by a nurse named Florence Nightingale.

_____ 2. Marie Curie was the first person to win two Nobel Prizes in two different fields.

_____ 3. The first woman to practice medicine in the United States with a degree was Emily Blackwell.

_____ 4. As of 2012, just over 47 percent of applicants to medical school were women.

_____ 5. CT scans use X-rays to take three-dimensional images of the insides of objects.

_____ 6. The Patient Protection and Affordable Care Act mandates a system that provides and offers health care coverage for all Americans.

_____ 7. The caduceus depicts two snakes wrapped around a healing staff.

_____ 8. In ancient times, most cultures believed shamans caused diseases and illnesses.

_____ 9. Traditional Chinese medicine was taught before classical Chinese medicine techniques were taught.

_____ 10. Edward Jenner was the first to employ modern anesthesia in 1842, when he used an ether-based anesthesia to remove a tumor from a patient's neck.

SHORT ANSWER

1. Explain why ether-based anesthesia was replaced with chloroform.

_____

_____

_____

_____

_____

2. Describe how Hungarian physician Ignaz Semmelweiss discovered the value of hand washing in health care.

_____

_____

_____

_____

3. Discuss the contributions to health care made by Pasteur.

_____

_____

_____

_____

4. Describe the invention of the first heart pacemaker, including how this invention improved over time.

_____

_____

_____

_____

5. Describe the Human Genome Project and its impact on medicine and medical care today.

_____

_____

_____

_____

6. Describe the American Medical Association milestones that have occurred since 2000.

_____

_____

_____

_____

7. Why was nursing not considered a respected profession in the 1850s?

_____

_____

_____

_____

© 2015 Pearson Education, Inc.

8. Explain the purpose of the World Health Organization.

_____

_____

_____

_____

_____

9. Discuss the philosophy behind evidence-based medicine.

_____

_____

_____

_____

_____

10. What are the mandates and goal of the Patient Protection and Affordable Care Act, also called Obamacare, as presented in this chapter of your student text?

_____

_____

_____

_____

_____

CHAPTER 2

Medical Assisting Certification and Scope of Practice

CHAPTER OUTLINE

Introduction

Educational Requirements of the Medical Assistant

The Medical Assistant's Scope of Practice

Certification Requirements for Other Allied Health Professionals

Review

COMPETENCY SKILLS PERFORMANCE

Procedure 2-1: Adapt to Change

CHAPTER REVIEW

- With dramatic changes occurring in health care including shorter hospital stays and managed care, physicians must rely on allied health care professionals, like medical assistants, to help care for patients.

- In coming years, the scope of medical assisting practice is expected to continue to grow and change. To practice according to local laws, medical assistants must know, and stay on top of, the legal parameters in their state.

- The types of certifications and registrations in the field dictate the educational requirements of medical assisting.

- Medical assisting recertification or registration can help the medical assistant stay abreast of industry developments and maintain the skills needed to remain competitive in the workplace.

- Professional organizations offer a number of benefits that are aimed at keeping the medical assistant optimally efficient and effective.

- Like the medical assisting profession, other allied health professions have created professional organizations to keep their members aligned and active.

LEARNING ACTIVITIES

To ensure that you have achieved the learning objectives in this chapter:

1. In the Terminology Review section on page 12, define the key terminology found in this chapter of your student text.

© 2015 Pearson Education, Inc.

2. List the benefits of becoming a certified or registered medical assistant.

_____

_____

_____

_____

_____

_____

_____

_____

3. List the professional organizations that certify or register medical assistants.

_____

_____

_____

_____

4. Describe the benefits of joining a professional medical assistant organization.

_____

_____

_____

_____

5. List the various professional associations that certify other allied health professionals, and include the type of health care professionals they certify.

_____

_____

_____

_____

_____

_____

_____

_____

_____

APPLIED LEARNING EXERCISES

Using a separate sheet of paper, complete the following assignments:

1. Review the educational requirements of the medical assistant as outlined in this chapter of your student text. Write a 1–2-page essay outlining the steps you will take to be successful in each of the classes you will take to become a medical assistant.

2. Using the Internet, look up the scope of practice for a medical assistant in your state. Write a 1–2-page essay that outlines the scope of medical assisting in your state.

TERMINOLOGY REVIEW

Using the glossary and highlighted terms in the textbook, define the following terms:

accredited: _____

_____

Accrediting Bureau of Health Education Schools (ABHES): _____

_____

administrative: _____

_____

American Medical Technologists (AMT): _____

_____

associate degree: _____

_____

certified medical assistant (CMA): _____

_____

clinical: _____

_____

Commission of Accreditation of Allied Health Education Programs (CAAHEP): _____

_____

community college: _____

_____

competency: _____

_____

practicum: _____

_____

proprietary school: _____

_____

recertification: _____

_____

registered medical assistant (RMA): _____

_____

© 2015 Pearson Education, Inc.

scope of practice: _____

_____

technical educational program: _____

_____

vocational program: _____

ABBREVIATIONS

Provide the meanings of the following abbreviations:

AAPC: _____

ABHES: _____

AHIMA: _____

AHDI: _____

AMT: _____

CAAHEP: _____

CCS: _____

CEU: _____

CLC: _____

CMA: _____

CMAA: _____

CMAS: _____

CMT: _____

COLT: _____

CPC: _____

CPR: _____

HIPAA: _____

LPN: _____

MLT: _____

MT: _____

NCCT: _____

NCMA: _____

NHA: _____

NP: _____

PA: _____

RMA: _____

RPT: _____

CRITICAL THINKING QUESTIONS

1. Wilma Rodriguez, RMA (AMT), is working as an administrative medical assistant in a large family practice clinic. Ron Lundberg is a medical assistant who has been working in this clinic for several years. Ron has not been through formal training as a medical assistant. One day, Ron notices Wilma performing a task he has not been trained to do. He asks her where she learned this task. Wilma explains the various courses she took as part of her formal training as a medical assistant. What courses would Wilma include in her response to Ron?

   _____

   _____

   _____

   _____

   _____

   _____

2. Krista Hernandez has finished all of the required classes in her medical assisting program. She is ready to begin her practicum. What are the requirements of a typical medical assisting practicum?

   _____

   _____

   _____

   _____

   _____

   _____

3. Shannon McLaren has just finished her training as an administrative medical assistant and is receiving her medical assisting certificate. She is trying to decide if she wants to obtain the Certified Medical Assistant (CMA [AAMA]) credential or the Registered Medical Assistant (RMA [AMT]) credential. She sits down to make a list of the similarities in the certification examination content outlines for the CMA (AAMA) and RMA (AMT) credentials. What administrative topic areas are included on each of these exams?

   _____

   _____

   _____

   _____

   _____

   _____

4. Diane Luder, CMA (AAMA), has been working as an administrative medical assistant in a busy pediatric office for 5 years. Diane's job has been in the billing and coding department. She is interested in becoming a certified coder. What organizations might she research for this credential?

   _____

   _____

   _____

   _____

   _____

   _____

© 2015 Pearson Education, Inc.

CHAPTER REVIEW TEST

MULTIPLE CHOICE

Circle the letter of the correct answer.

1. The American Health Information Management Association is a national organization of professionals who work in which of the following fields?
   a. Medical records
   b. Coding
   c. Health information management
   d. Medical transcription
   e. a, b, and c

2. AAPC offers a voluntary credentialing program with examinations that confer which of the following?
   a. CPC
   b. COLT
   c. MLT
   d. CMA (AAMA)
   e. RMA (AMT)

3. The American Medical Technologists offers certification or registration as which of the following?
   a. RMA
   b. CPC
   c. CMA
   d. NCMA
   e. All of the above

4. Currently, medical assistants must work under the direction and supervision of which of the following health care professionals?
   a. Physicians
   b. Nurse practitioners
   c. Physician assistants
   d. Medical coders
   e. a, b, and c

5. Joining a professional association for medical assistants offers which of the following benefits to the medical assistant?
   a. Opportunity to earn continuing education credits
   b. Access to information on laws relating credits to the profession
   c. Group insurance plans
   d. Subscriptions to professional journals
   e. All of the above

6. Which of the following is a requirement for medical assistants who wish to sit for the RMA (AMT) exam?
   a. Be at least 21 years of age
   b. Have at least 1 year of experience working as a medical assistant
   c. Be a graduate of an accredited medical assisting program
   d. Be a certified medical coder
   e. All of the above

7. In addition to the RMA (registered medical assistant) and CMAS (certified medical administrative specialist) certification, the AMT offers certification or registration as a(n) _____.

    a. MT (medical technologist)

    b. MLT (medical laboratory technician)

    c. COLT (certified office laboratory consultant)

    d. RPT (registered phlebotomy technician)

    e. All of the above

8. In order to maintain certified medical assisting CMA (AAMA) status, medical assistants must complete recertification every _____ years.

    a. 2

    b. 3

    c. 4

    d. 5

    e. 6

9. Which of the following organizations was established as part of an effort to achieve recognition for the medical transcription profession?

    a. The American Health Information Management Association

    b. The Association for Healthcare Documentation Integrity

    c. The American Medical Technologists

    d. The American Academy of Professional Coders

    e. None of the above

10. In coming years, the scope of practice in medical assisting is expected to _____.

    a. remain the same

    b. decline

    c. expand

    d. include administrative competencies only

    e. include clinical competencies only

TRUE/FALSE

Identify whether the statement is true (T) or false (F).

_____ 1. Medical assisting certification is mandatory.

_____ 2. In many states, many malpractice insurance carriers offer discounts to physicians who employ only certified medical assistants.

_____ 3. Certification or registration means medical assistants have been trained to a standard required by the AAMA.

_____ 4. All accredited medical assisting programs include training on Health Insurance Portability and Accountability Act (HIPAA) regulations.

_____ 5. The scope of medical assisting practice is expected to remain the same in the coming years.

_____ 6. The AAMA offers certification as a medical administrative specialist.

_____ 7. Accredited medical assisting programs must teach in all areas of the AAMA Occupational Analysis, including administrative, clinical, and general skills.

_____ 8. Medical assistants can perform venipuncture in all states.

_____ 9. Medical assisting is currently a licensed profession.

_____ 10. Accredited medical assisting programs may be found in community colleges.

© 2015 Pearson Education, Inc.

SHORT ANSWER

1. Explain the purpose of the AAMA Occupational Analysis.

   _____

   _____

   _____

   _____

2. List two reasons why a physician would want to hire a certified or registered medical assistant over a medical assistant who has not received any formal medical training.

   _____

   _____

   _____

   _____

3. List the eight statements included in the Medical Assistant's Creed.

   _____

   _____

   _____

   _____

4. List 10 classes that would be taught within an accredited medical assisting program.

   _____

   _____

   _____

   _____

5. What are two benefits of the practicum from the student's point of view?

   _____

   _____

   _____

   _____

6. What is HIPAA, and why are HIPAA training and compliance mandated for all health care professionals?

   _____

   _____

   _____

   _____

7. What are the requirements to sit for the RMA (AMT) certification exam?

_____

_____

_____

_____

_____

8. In addition to the RMA (AMT) and CMAS (AMT) certifications, what other certifications are offered by the American Medical Technologists (AMT)?

_____

_____

_____

_____

9. When a patient incorrectly identifies the medical assistant as a nurse, how should the medical assistant respond?

_____

_____

_____

_____

_____

_____

_____

_____

10. What are the differences between a community college and a technical education/vocational program?

_____

_____

_____

_____

_____

© 2015 Pearson Education, Inc.

CHAPTER 3
Roles and Responsibilities of the Health Care Team

CHAPTER OUTLINE

CHAPTER REVIEW

- Medical assistants are highly skilled medical professionals who are considered a vital part of the health care team. They work closely with physicians, nurses, pharmacists, physical therapists, and insurance specialists, among others.

- Today's medical assistants have typically received formal education in an accredited medical assisting program and have been trained to perform a variety of administrative as well as clinical tasks.

- Medical assisting is a career with multiple responsibilities, and it requires a set of unique qualities, including, but not limited to, loyalty, empathy, dependability, and flexibility. Like all members of the health care team, medical assistants must understand the value of respecting patient confidentiality and of proper communication with the patients they work with.

- The most important part of the medical assistant's job is to act as the patient's advocate. Because patients will likely spend more time with the medical assistant than with the physician, it is extremely important for the medical assistant to develop a rapport with patients.

- Medical assistants should practice good personal hygiene for their body and their clothing. Artificial nails should not be worn on the job. Medical assistants should also avoid wearing excessive or obtrusive jewelry. Body piercings, except for posts in the ear lobes, should not be visible, and tattoos and other body art should be covered during office hours. Hair should be clean and pulled back, and scented lotions and perfumes should be minimized out of consideration for patients with allergies. Uniforms, including shoes, should be clean and in good repair. The medical assistant's nametag should be in plain view and clearly identify the name and role of the medical assistant. Policies for dress, jewelry, hairstyles, piercings, and tattoos will vary from office to office, so medical assistants should review these policies when they are hired.

- Efficient time management requires strong organizational skills. A time-management journal is an effective tool for medical assistants to use to help prioritize projects and manage their time effectively.

- Career opportunities for the medical assistant exist in a variety of settings, including ambulatory care settings and insurance companies. The growing nature of the industry will continue to offer medical assistants new and varied career opportunities with other members of the health care profession.

© 2015 Pearson Education, Inc.

- Today's health care team is multidisciplinary, which means that many different types of providers and medical specialists help provide a patient's care. Medical assistants should have a good working knowledge of the types of care these professionals provide so they can accurately relay information to patients when doctors make referrals, as well as direct patients to the appropriate members of the health care team.

LEARNING ACTIVITIES

To ensure that you have achieved the learning objectives in this chapter:

1. In the Terminology Review section on page 21, define the key terminology found in this chapter of your student text.

2. After reading through this chapter of your student textbook, create a list of the desirable qualities of a medical assistant. Describe the qualities you feel you have that will benefit you in a career as a medical assistant.

_____

_____

_____

_____

_____

3. Describe the proper attire of the medical assistant in the work setting.

_____

_____

_____

_____

_____

4. Create a list of the other members of the health care team as discussed in your student text. Describe the role of each of these health care professionals.

_____

_____

_____

_____

_____

_____

_____

5. List and describe five medical practice specializations discussed in this chapter of your student text.

_____

_____

© 2015 Pearson Education, Inc.

_____
_____
_____
_____
_____
_____
_____
_____
_____
_____
_____
_____

APPLIED LEARNING EXERCISES

Using a separate sheet of paper, complete the following assignments:

1. Write an essay that outlines various techniques for improving time-management skills.
2. Using the Internet and a local newspaper, create a list of current career opportunities available to the medical assistant in your area.
3. Choose one of the types of complementary and alternative medicine listed in Table 3-6 of the student text. Research a provider who works in your area practicing in this specialty. What type of care does he or she provide?

TERMINOLOGY REVIEW

Using a dictionary and highlighted terms in the textbook, define the following terms:

accredited: _____
_____

administrative skills: _____
_____

advocate: _____
_____

ambulatory care centers: _____
_____

attitude: _____
_____

body language: _____
_____

clinical skills: _____
_____

confidentiality: _____

_____

courtesy: _____

_____

credibility: _____

_____

dependability: _____

_____

empathy: _____

_____

flexibility: _____

_____

initiative: _____

_____

loyalty: _____

_____

multidisciplinary: _____

_____

rapport: _____

_____

respect: _____

_____

ABBREVIATIONS

Provide the meanings of the following abbreviations:

ACPE: _____

ADN: _____

AMA: _____

ASCP: _____

BSN: _____

CAM: _____

DO: _____

DEA: _____

DME: _____

FDA: _____

HIPAA: _____

HUC: _____

© 2015 Pearson Education, Inc.

LPN: _____

LVN: _____

MD: _____

MLT: _____

MPJE: _____

NAPLEX: _____

NP: _____

OTC: _____

PA: _____

PT: _____

PTA: _____

RN: _____

CRITICAL THINKING QUESTIONS

1. Marla Darlunberg is the medical office manager at the Mountain View Health Clinic. She is in the process of hiring a new administrative medical assistant. What qualities should Marla look for in a candidate?

_____

_____

_____

_____

_____

2. Roger Powell, CMA (AAMA), is the administrative medical assistant at a family medical practice in his community. Because he works in the same community in which he lives, he often runs into patients while doing everyday tasks such as walking his dog, shopping, or running errands. One day, on his way to the bank, Roger runs into a patient who asks him for specific information regarding the health care of another patient. How should Roger respond?

_____

_____

_____

_____

_____

3. Wanda Rolen, CMA (AAMA), is working with Dr. Brockman, a naturopathic physician. Wanda notices that Dr. Brockman frequently prescribes complementary alternative medicine techniques to her patients. Wanda is talking to her neighbor about the use of complementary alternative medicine and finds that the neighbor is unfamiliar with these therapies. How can Wanda describe what complementary alternative medicine is and why patients might seek this type of care?

_____

_____

_____

_____

_____

4. Yelena Rubashka is taking an administrative class as part of her medical assistant training. She has been given an assignment to create a list of the common medical specialties patients will seek care with. What specialties should Yelena include in her list, and how should she describe them?

_____

_____

_____

_____

_____

5. James Dugan has nearly completed his training in a medical assisting program. He is considering continuing in his education in order to pursue a nursing degree. What type of education would James have if he pursued a nursing degree?

_____

_____

_____

_____

_____

CHAPTER REVIEW TEST

MULTIPLE CHOICE

Circle the letter of the correct answer.

1. Which of the following locations is one where a nurse might work?
   a. Home health care
   b. Hospitals
   c. Insurance companies
   d. a, b, and c
   e. None of the above

2. Many physician assistant (PA) programs require at least _____ years of college and some health care experience before admission.
   a. 2
   b. 3
   c. 4
   d. 5
   e. 6

3. Education programs for pharmacists require at least _____ years of college.
   a. 3
   b. 4
   c. 5
   d. 6
   e. 7

                                                © 2015 Pearson Education, Inc.

4. In the United States, physicians must attend _____ years of medical school.
   a. 4
   b. 5
   c. 6
   d. 7
   e. 8

5. Which of the following guidelines will help the medical assistant maintain a professional image?
   a. Do not discuss personal problems while in the workplace.
   b. Avoid participating in gossip in the workplace.
   c. Do not conduct personal business during work hours.
   d. Do not procrastinate.
   e. All of the above

6. Which of the following projects a professional image for the medical assistant?
   a. Long hair
   b. Artificial nails
   c. Tasteful nose ring
   d. Clean uniform
   e. All of the above

7. Which of the following is true of the professional medical assistant's image?
   a. Medical assistants should practice good personal hygiene for their body and their clothing.
   b. Artificial nails may harbor bacteria and should not be worn on the job.
   c. Medical assistants should avoid wearing excessive or obtrusive jewelry, because hands will be washed and gloves donned several times a day.
   d. Body piercings, except for posts in the ear lobes, should not be visible.
   e. All of the above

8. Which of the following cultures believes showing an open mouth, as when yawning, is considered rude?
   a. Asian-Pacific
   b. Chinese
   c. Japanese
   d. Korean
   e. Arabic

9. Which of the following cultures uses bowing as a traditional greeting?
   a. Asian-Pacific
   b. Chinese
   c. Japanese
   d. Korean
   e. Arabic

10. Which of the following is considered unprofessional when done in patients' view?
   a. Eating
   b. Using the telephone
   c. Speaking with coworkers
   d. Remaining calm and polite
   e. All of the above

TRUE/FALSE

Identify whether the statement is true (T) or false (F).

_____ 1. Medical assistants should never release patient information without a patient's written authorization or a court order.

_____ 2. Medical assistants should be familiar with the prevailing cultural customs in their areas.

_____ 3. Medical assistants should keep their personal beliefs separate from patient care.

_____ 4. Patients may stop seeing their physician if they feel uncomfortable with the office staff.

_____ 5. In a large office, medical assisting duties are often more specialized.

_____ 6. The professional standard for the medical assistant does not extend to social media sites, such as Facebook or Twitter.

_____ 7. Complementary alternative medicine is a growing alternative to traditional medical techniques.

_____ 8. Since medical assistants are only responsible for their own scope of practice, it is not important for the MA to understand the roles and responsibilities of other members of the health care team.

_____ 9. Medical assistants might find employment working for insurance companies.

_____ 10. One of the keys to efficient time management in the medical office is having good organizational skills.

SHORT ANSWER

1. List five duties of the clinical medical assistant and five duties of the administrative medical assistant.

_____

_____

_____

_____

_____

2. What is the difference between empathy and sympathy?

_____

_____

_____

_____

_____

3. Why is it important for the medical assistant to have an understanding of the various complementary alternative medical therapies commonly used?

_____

_____

_____

_____

_____

4. How much money is spent in the United States for complementary alternative medicine each year? Does that revenue typically come from patients or their insurance carriers? Explain.

_____

_____

_____

_____

5. Outline various complementary and alternative medicine therapies described in this chapter, including their treatment objective.

_____

_____

© 2015 Pearson Education, Inc.

_____

_____

_____

6. How does the nurse practitioner differ from the physician's assistant?

_____

_____

_____

_____

7. Describe the role of the pharmacist as part of the health care team.

_____

_____

_____

_____

8. What is meant by the term *multidisciplinary* with regard to the health care team?

_____

_____

_____

_____

9. Explain the role of the physician assistant in the medical office.

_____

_____

_____

_____

10. Where might a medical assistant find employment?

_____

_____

_____

_____

© 2015 Pearson Education, Inc.

CHAPTER 4
Medicine and the Law

CHAPTER OUTLINE

COMPETENCY SKILLS PERFORMANCE

© 2015 Pearson Education, Inc.

CHAPTER REVIEW

- Medical assistants face many situations that involve medical law. Each state has unique laws governing health care and the medical assisting profession. It is crucial for the medical assistant to know the laws of his or her state and to uphold those laws at all times. Since laws can change over time, medical assistants must keep abreast of these changes and understand how these changes may need to be implemented in the medical setting.

- Tort law deals with situations in which someone has been injured by another's actions or inactions. Torts are one of two types: unintentional or intentional. An unintentional tort occurs when a mistake is made. The vast majority of medical malpractice cases fall into this category, because unintentional torts usually involve negligence.

- Medical assistants, as part of the health care team, are integral in making certain that patients understand procedures the physician orders. Though obtaining consent is the duty of the physician, the medical assistant is often part of the consent process, from helping to explain the procedure to going over the necessary paperwork involved.

- Health care providers are human, and sometimes mistakes are made. When these mistakes lead to patient injury, malpractice lawsuits may be filed. Medical assistants need to have a solid understanding of how to prevent medical malpractice and actively look for ways to prevent patient injury.

- Physicians have various public duties they must perform as part of their practice. These duties include reporting suspected abuse and vaccine injuries. Medical assistants are frequently part of the process of reporting these cases.

- Physicians and patients both have duties they should uphold in the physician-patient relationship. Many of these are dictated by law, especially the physicians' responsibilities.

- A contract is an agreement between two or more parties that the law will recognize. Contracts in health care surround the consent for care and payment for services rendered. Physicians and patients operate using two types of contracts: (1) implied and (2) expressed.

- The doctor-patient contract is typically resolved once the patient has completed the prescribed course of treatment outlined by the physician. While the patient may choose to end the doctor-patient relationship at any time, the physician must follow legal protocol to end the relationship.

- Medical assistants are called upon to oversee the release of patient medical records. Strict attention to the laws relating to patient confidentiality is of the utmost importance when copying and releasing patient medical records. These laws are more strict with regard to some areas of medical records, such as HIV/AIDS, mental illness, and family planning. The Health Insurance Portability and Accountability Act (HIPAA) is a law that outlines how patient personal information is to be kept confidential.

- The Good Samaritan Act protects health care workers from being sued when they voluntarily render assistance in emergency situations.

- The Patient Care Partnership outlines patients' expectations, rights, and responsibilities while in the hospital setting and explains the quality of care the patient can expect to receive, recognizing that a clean and safe environment should be provided to all patients.

- Monitoring agencies, such as The Joint Commission (TJC) and the Occupational Safety and Health Administration (OSHA), provide rules and regulations that protect the safety of patients as well as employees in the health care setting.

- Today, many patients use advance directives to outline their wishes should they be unable to speak for themselves. Advance directives consist of living wills, orders outlining patients' desire to not be resuscitated, and durable power of attorney for health care.

- Title VII of the Civil Rights Act of 1964 was passed to protect employees from discrimination in the workplace. Under this act, employers cannot refuse to hire, refuse to equally compensate, or fire an employee based on race, color, sex, religion, or national origin.

© 2015 Pearson Education, Inc.

- The Controlled Substances Act of 1970 regulates the manufacture, distribution, and dispensing of narcotics and nonnarcotic drugs that are considered to have a high potential for abuse.

LEARNING ACTIVITIES

To ensure that you have achieved the learning objectives in this chapter:

1. In the Terminology Review section on page 32, define the key terminology found in this chapter of your student text.

2. Describe criminal law and civil law.

_____

_____

_____

_____

_____

_____

_____

_____

_____

3. Describe a situation where a signed consent form would be required.

_____

_____

_____

_____

_____

_____

4. Describe a situation where implied consent would be sufficient.

_____

_____

_____

_____

5. Create a list of the ways in which an administrative medical assistant helps to maintain patient confidentiality.

_____

_____

_____

_____

_____

_____

© 2015 Pearson Education, Inc.

6. Create a list of the various federal and local regulatory organizations that oversee health care clinics in your state. Include the qualities health care professionals need to comply with these agencies' regulations.

_____

_____

_____

_____

_____

_____

_____

_____

_____

7. Using the Internet as a research source, find out if your state has a Patients' Bill of Rights. If so, what is included?

_____

_____

_____

_____

_____

8. Create a list of the monitoring agencies that oversee ambulatory health care clinics.

_____

_____

_____

_____

_____

APPLIED LEARNING EXERCISES

Using a separate sheet of paper, complete the following assignments:

1. Using the Internet as a research source, search for a malpractice case. Describe the case you find and include whether the patient or the physician won the case. Did you feel the case was decided fairly? Why or why not?

2. Using the Internet as a research source, create a list of the physician's public duties in your state.

3. Using the Internet as a research source, write an essay describing the history of HIPAA and how that law affects ambulatory care clinics.

4. Using the Internet as a research source, determine if your state has a list of conditions and diseases that must be reported to local, county, or state agencies. If it does, list the mandatory requirements for five of the conditions or diseases.

TERMINOLOGY REVIEW

Using the glossary and highlighted terms in the textbook, define the following terms:

administrative law: _____

_____

advance directives: _____

_____

appeal: _____

_____

assault: _____

_____

assumption of risk: _____

_____

battery: _____

_____

civil law: _____

_____

commercial law: _____

_____

common law: _____

_____

comparative negligence: _____

_____

conscience clauses: _____

_____

constitutional law: _____

_____

contract law: _____

_____

contributory negligence: _____

_____

criminal law: _____

_____

damages: _____

_____

defamation of character: _____

_____

discovery rule: _____

_____

© 2015 Pearson Education, Inc.

duress: _____

_____

expert witness: _____

_____

expressed consent: _____

_____

expressed contract: _____

_____

Family Medical Leave Act (FMLA): _____

_____

felony: _____

_____

Four Ds of Negligence: _____

_____

fraud: _____

_____

Good Samaritan Act: _____

_____

Health Insurance Portability and Accountability Act (HIPAA): _____

_____

immunity: _____

_____

implied consent: _____

_____

implied contract: _____

_____

informed consent: _____

_____

intentional tort: _____

_____

international law: _____

_____

invasion of privacy: _____

_____

malfeasance: _____

_____

malpractice: _____

_____

malpractice insurance policy: _____

_____

misdemeanor: _____

_____

misfeasance: _____

_____

negligence: _____

_____

nonfeasance: _____

_____

Patient Care Partnership: _____

_____

portability: _____

_____

precedent: _____

_____

protected health information: _____

_____

regulatory law: _____

_____

res ipsa loquitur: _____

_____

res judicata: _____

_____

respondeat superior: _____

_____

settled: _____

_____

standard of care: _____

_____

statute of limitations: _____

_____

subpoena: _____

_____

subpoena duces tecum: _____

_____

tort law: _____

_____

© 2015 Pearson Education, Inc.

undue influence: _____

_____

unintentional tort: _____

_____

ABBREVIATIONS

Provide the meanings of the following abbreviations:

AAMA: _____

ADA: _____

AHA: _____

AHIMA: _____

AIDS: _____

CDC: _____

CLIA: _____

CMS: _____

CPR: _____

DEA: _____

DNR: _____

EIN: _____

FDA: _____

FMLA: _____

HIPAA: _____

HIV: _____

IRS: _____

MSA: _____

OSHA: _____

PHI: _____

STI: _____

TJC: _____

CRITICAL THINKING QUESTIONS

1. Ian Rairdon is a certified medical assistant in Dr. Robinson's office. As a health care provider who dispenses, administers, and prescribes controlled substances to his patients, Dr. Robinson has asked Ian to register him with the DEA. What law regulates the manufacture, distribution, and dispensing of narcotic and nonnarcotic drugs that are considered to have a high potential for abuse? Why must Ian register Dr. Robinson with the DEA?

_____

_____

_____

_____

2. Gregory Chan, CMA (AAMA), has been asked by his office manager to create an outline of the clinic's OSHA exposure control plan. What information will Gregory need to include in this outline?

_____

_____

_____

_____

_____

3. Janice Andrews, RMA (AMT), is collecting an elderly patient's insurance card upon the patient's arrival to the medical office. When the patient asks Janice about the reputation of the cardiology practice located across the street, Janice responds by saying, "I would not recommend that you see that cardiologist; I hear he has a drinking problem." Could this statement be grounds for a lawsuit? Why or why not? What type of intentional tort has Janice committed?

_____

_____

_____

_____

_____

4. Mr. Henderson, a patient in the South Shore Medical Clinic, is discussing his concerns regarding his upcoming surgery with the registered medical assistant. Mr. Henderson asks the medical assistant how he might outline his wishes in the event he is unable to speak for himself after his surgery. What information should the medical assistant include in her response to Mr. Henderson?

_____

_____

_____

_____

5. Anthony Martinez is a certified medical assistant at the Rosemont Medical Clinic. Mr. Jeremy Frank, a patient in the medical office, has requested a copy of his medical record. What is the proper procedure Anthony must follow for the release of Mr. Frank's personal patient information in order to ensure the release does not violate HIPAA regulations?

_____

_____

_____

_____

_____

© 2015 Pearson Education, Inc.

CHAPTER REVIEW TEST

MULTIPLE CHOICE

Circle the letter of the correct answer.

1. In many states, OSHA dictates that any employee who is exposed to bodily fluids in the workplace must be given a _____ vaccine free of charge.
   a. hepatitis A
   b. hepatitis B
   c. hepatitis C
   d. HIV
   e. smallpox

2. The American Hospital Association first adopted a Patients' Bill of Rights in _____.
   a. 1962
   b. 1972
   c. 1982
   d. 1992
   e. 2001

3. _____ is legislation derived from the Old English legal system that is based on precedence.
   a. Common law
   b. Commercial law
   c. Constitutional law
   d. Contract law
   e. Criminal law

4. The Americans with Disabilities laws apply to employers with _____ or more employees.
   a. 5
   b. 10
   c. 15
   d. 20
   e. 25

5. Which of the following is prohibited under Title VII of the Civil Rights Act of 1964?
   a. An employer firing an employee based on race
   b. An employer refusing to hire an employee based on religion
   c. An employer refusing to equally compensate medical assistants with the same educational background and experience
   d. An employer firing an employee based on national origin
   e. All of the above

6. Living wills are legal in _____ state(s).
   a. 1
   b. 15
   c. 35
   d. 45
   e. every

© 2015 Pearson Education, Inc.

7. The general penalty for the failure to comply with HIPAA requirements and standards is
_____.

a. $100–$50,000 if the violation occurred due to ignorance of the law
b. $1,000–$50,000 for violations considered reasonable cause
c. $10,000–$50,000 for violations considered due to willful neglect, where the violator corrected the actions
d. $50,000 for violations due to willful neglect, where the violator did not correct the actions
e. All of the above

8. HIPAA Business Associate agreements should be signed by which of following?

a. Equipment repair persons
b. Software support technicians
c. A medical assistant performing a practicum in the clinic
d. Cleaning staff
e. All of the above

9. The Health Insurance Portability and Accountability Act (HIPAA) of 1996 was enacted to reform health care by _____.

a. improving portability and continuity in group and individual insurance
b. combatting waste, fraud, and abuse in health insurance and health care delivery
c. promoting the use of medical savings accounts (MSAs)
d. improving access to long-term care services and coverage
e. All of the above

10. Which of the following is NOT true of super-protected health information?

a. Super-protected information includes material pertaining to HIV testing.
b. Super-protected information includes material pertaining to STI treatment.
c. Super-protected information can be released to a third party without separate authorization.
d. Super-protected information cannot be released without a specific request from the patient.
e. Super-protected information includes information pertaining to mental illness.

TRUE/FALSE

Identify whether the statement is true (T) or false (F).

_____ 1. Minor patients may receive copies of any part of their own medical records.

_____ 2. In many states, children under the age of 18 may receive treatment for certain types of conditions without parental consent.

_____ 3. Medical records may never be released without the patient's written consent.

_____ 4. In rare cases, medical offices may release original patient records.

_____ 5. Medical assistants cannot release information to the patient's health insurance company without that patient's consent.

© 2015 Pearson Education, Inc.

_____ 6. The Good Samaritan Act protects health care workers from being sued when they render first aid in emergency situations outside the health care setting.

_____ 7. If a physician wishes to terminate the physician-patient relationship, the physician must give the patient 90 days to find another physician.

_____ 8. A contract does not need to be written to be valid.

_____ 9. Expressed contracts are those that are always spoken.

_____ 10. Implied contracts are those that are always written.

SHORT ANSWER

1. Under what circumstances might a physician have his or her license to practice medicine revoked?

_____
_____
_____
_____
_____

2. What process that should be followed for reporting vaccine injuries?

_____
_____
_____
_____

3. Explain how capping the money awarded to a patient injured by medical malpractice may well cost taxpayers money with regard to the cost of caring for the injured patient.

_____
_____
_____
_____
_____

4. Describe what an "expert witness" is with regard to a medical malpractice lawsuit.

_____
_____
_____
_____

5. What is the "standard of care" as it pertains to a medical malpractice lawsuit?

_____
_____
_____
_____

6. Define the Latin phrases "res judicata" and "res ipsa loquitur," and describe how each of these phrases pertains to a medical malpractice lawsuit.

_____

_____

_____

_____

_____

7. Describe the statute of limitations period as it pertains to medical malpractice in the state where you live.

_____

_____

_____

_____

_____

8. Define the three types of medical malpractice awards.

_____

_____

_____

_____

_____

9. Define the Four Ds of Negligence.

_____

_____

_____

_____

_____

10. Define the doctrine of respondeat superior, and explain how it pertains to the actions of the medical assistant working for a physician in a medical office.

_____

_____

_____

_____

_____

© 2015 Pearson Education, Inc.

CHAPTER 5
Medicine and Ethics

CHAPTER OUTLINE

Introduction

History of Ethics in Medicine

Ethical Considerations

Ethical Model

Raising Ethical Issues in Health Care

Bioethics

Clinical Research

Employer-Mandated Medical Care

Review

CHAPTER REVIEW

- Ethics in medicine has evolved over time and continues to evolve today. Medical ethics pertain to health care professionals acting only within their legal scope of practice.

- The concepts surrounding medical ethics have been around since the time of Hippocrates, a classical Greek physician who lived between 460 and 377 B.C.E. The Hippocratic Oath was the first basic guide for medical ethics.

- Medical ethics govern the behavior of health care professionals. Every professional association has its own code of ethics that details the actions that are considered ethical by that profession. The American Association of Medical Assistants (AAMA) has a Code of Ethics that addresses areas the medical assistant must strive to adhere to. Since 1999, the AAMA has had a policy of sanctioning medical assistants who violate its disciplinary standards.

- Medical assistants are legally bound by law and scope of practice to treat patients lawfully and ethically and to document correctly in patients' charts. If medical assistants wonder whether actions cross ethical or legal boundaries, they can use ethical decision-making models to assist in making decisions in the health care field.

- The American Medical Association outlines several ethical issues that pertain to ethics in the management of patient care and finances in the health care setting.

- Medical bioethics addresses areas that affect human life and includes topics such as abortion, abuse, allocation of health resources, artificial insemination, infertility treatments, stem cell research, surrogacy, cloning, genetic counseling, physician-assisted suicide, organ donation, and treating patients with HIV/AIDS.

- Clinical research typically consists of researchers studying the effects of a medicine or treatment on a particular disease or condition. Clinical research is seen by some as an ethical issue because harm may be caused rather than benefit.

© 2015 Pearson Education, Inc.

- Many health care employers today mandate that their employees receive certain types of medical care as a condition of employment. Most often, this care consists of vaccinations against a variety of illnesses and diseases.

LEARNING ACTIVITIES

To ensure that you have achieved the learning objectives in this chapter:

1. In the Terminology Review section on page 43, define the key terminology found in this chapter of your student text.

2. List key events in the history of ethics in medicine, and describe how these events impact medical care today.

_____

_____

_____

_____

_____

_____

_____

_____

3. What are the implications for a medical assistant who performs outside his or her scope of practice?

_____

_____

_____

_____

_____

4. When faced with an ethical dilemma, what questions, based on the Blanchard and Peale Ethical Model, might medical assistants ask themselves to determine if their actions will cross ethical or legal boundaries?

_____

_____

_____

_____

_____

5. The American Medical Association (AMA) has outlined several ethical issues pertaining to the management of patient care in particular areas, including organ transplantation, clinical research, and obstetrics. What are the specific guidelines outlined by the AMA with regard to these three areas?

_____

_____

_____

© 2015 Pearson Education, Inc.

_____

_____

_____

APPLIED LEARNING EXERCISES

Using a separate sheet of paper, complete the following assignments:

1. Look up the professional Code of Ethics on the AAMA Web site. Describe what the professional Code of Ethics is for medical assistants, and explain why it is important for medical assistants to have one.

2. Using the Internet as a research source, find a news story that includes a medical ethical or bioethical issue. Describe the story, and include how you feel about the situation described in the story.

TERMINOLOGY REVIEW

Using the glossary and highlighted terms in the textbook, define the following terms:

abuse: _____

_____

artificial insemination: _____

_____

bioethics: _____

_____

cloning: _____

_____

medical ethics: _____

_____

morals: _____

_____

values: _____

_____

ABBREVIATIONS

Provide the meanings of the following abbreviations:

AAMA: _____

AI: _____

CMA: _____

CRITICAL THINKING QUESTIONS

1. Ronnie Wilkins, RMA (AMT), is working with Mr. Martin Guzman, a 42-year-old patient. Mr. Guzman has asked Ronnie if she knows how he can go about becoming an organ donor. What information should Ronnie include in her explanation of the laws pertaining to organ donation? Why is organ donation considered a bioethical issue?

_____

_____

_____

_____

_____

2. Beth Clark is taking an administrative medical assisting course as part of her medical assisting training. She has been given the assignment of writing a paper that outlines the current ethical standpoints of the AMA. What points should Beth include?

_____

_____

_____

_____

_____

3. A client infected with HIV is scheduled to visit a busy family medical practice. From an ethical standpoint, why is it important for the medical staff to treat this patient?

_____

_____

_____

_____

_____

4. Ms. Andrea Kindle is awaiting a kidney transplant. She understands that every year, approximately 6,000 Americans die waiting for organ transplants. Ms. Kindle confides in the medical assistant that she is willing to pay a considerable amount of money for a kidney. What information should the medical assistant provide Ms. Kindle with regard to financial compensation and organ donation?

_____

_____

_____

_____

_____

CHAPTER REVIEW TEST

MULTIPLE CHOICE

Circle the letter of the correct answer.

1. Which of the following is considered the first basic guide for medical ethics?
   a. Nuremberg Code
   b. Declaration of Helsinski
   c. Hippocratic Oath
   d. AAMA Code of Ethics
   e. AMA Code of Ethics

© 2015 Pearson Education, Inc.

2. The _____ outlined 10 points regarding permissible experimentation on human beings.
   a. Nuremberg Code
   b. Declaration of Helsinski
   c. Hippocratic Oath
   d. AAMA Code of Ethics
   e. AMA Code of Ethics

3. The _____ concentrates on human subjects of research studies and covers ethical guidelines for the medical profession, including well-informed subjects and a focus on the safety and well-being of those involved.
   a. Nuremberg Code
   b. Declaration of Helsinski
   c. Hippocratic Oath
   d. AAMA Code of Ethics
   e. AMA Code of Ethics

4. The American Association of Medical Assistants (AAMA) includes which of the following in its Code of Ethics?
   a. Rendering services with respect for human dignity
   b. Respecting patient confidentiality, except when the law requires information
   c. Upholding the honor and high principles set forth by the AAMA
   d. Continually improving knowledge and skills for the benefit of patients and the health care team
   e. All of the above

5. Which of the following questions is NOT based on the Blanchard and Peale Ethical Model?
   a. Is the action ethical?
   b. Is the action legal?
   c. How will the action make me feel?
   d. Will I be compensated for this action?
   e. How would I feel if the action, and my involvement, was published in the local newspaper?

6. Which of the following statements represents the American Medical Association's (AMA's) ethical stance on organ transplantation?
   a. Physicians must consider age when deciding who gets the organ.
   b. Priority must be given to the patient who has the strongest chance of obtaining long-term benefit.
   c. Physicians must consider a person's individual worth to society when deciding who gets the organ.
   d. Financial compensation may be made for organ donation.
   e. None of the above

7. _____ pertains to a family undergoing a health history and a discussion of their ethnic makeup prior to conception.
   a. Surrogacy
   b. Abortion
   c. Genetic counseling
   d. Artificial insemination
   e. None of the above

8. Which of the following types of abuse is defined as the illegal taking, misuse, or concealment of funds or property of a vulnerable adult or child?
   a. Exploitation
   b. Abandonment
   c. Neglect
   d. Physical abuse
   e. Emotional abuse

9. _____ is defined as the failure of a caregiver, parent, or guardian to provide food, shelter, health care, or protection to the person being cared for.
   a. Emotional abuse
   b. Exploitation
   c. Physical abuse
   d. Emotional abuse
   e. Neglect

10. Which of the following statements represents the AMA's ethical stance on finances in the health care setting?
   a. Patient care should be dictated by the patient's ability to pay.
   b. Physicians can charge for missed appointments under any circumstances.
   c. Physicians can withhold the medical record from the patient if the patient has an outstanding bill.
   d. Physicians cannot charge interest on medical bills under any circumstances.
   e. Fees for service must be reasonable, fair, and based on Current Procedural Terminology (CPT) code guidelines regarding the nature of the care involved.

TRUE/FALSE

Identify whether the statement is true (T) or false (F).

_____ 1. Medical law governs the behavior of health care professionals.

_____ 2. The American Association of Medical Assistants created the first basic guide for medical ethics.

_____ 3. The Nuremberg Code contained 10 points regarding permissible experimentation on human beings.

_____ 4. It is illegal for the medical assistant to perform outside his or her scope of practice, even when the physician requests and specifically trains the MA to complete a particular task.

_____ 5. Medical assistants can use the Blanchard and Peale Ethical Model to determine if their actions will cross ethical or legal boundaries.

_____ 6. Neglect is the illegal taking, misuse, or concealment of funds or property of a vulnerable adult or a child.

_____ 7. Exploitation is the failure of a caregiver, parent, or guardian to provide food, shelter, health care, or protection to the person being cared for.

_____ 8. Physicians are not responsible for reporting sexual abuse to the local law enforcement agency.

_____ 9. Domestic violence can take many forms, including emotional, sexual, and physical abuse and threats of abuse.

_____ 10. Stem cell research is considered a bioethical issue because embryos must be destroyed in order to perform embryonic stem cell research.

SHORT ANSWER

1. Describe the ethical guidelines of the Nuremberg Code.

_____

_____

 © 2015 Pearson Education, Inc.

_____

_____

2. The American Association of Medical Assistants (AAMA) has a code of ethics that addresses five areas the medical assistant must strive for. What are these five areas?

_____

_____

_____

_____

_____

3. Provide three examples of activities or lifestyle differences the medical assistant may face when working with patients and/or coworkers.

_____

_____

_____

_____

_____

4. Describe the different forms of abuse, including physical, emotional, and sexual.

_____

_____

_____

_____

_____

5. Define the terms _neglect, exploitation,_ and _abandonment._

_____

_____

_____

_____

_____

6. Why is stem cell research considered a bioethical issue?

_____

_____

_____

_____

7. Why is abortion considered a bioethical issue?

_____

_____

_____

_____

8. How are women treated for infertility?

_____

_____

_____

_____

_____

9. Why is in vitro fertilization considered a bioethical issue?

_____

_____

_____

_____

_____

10. Describe the different types of surrogacy, and explain why surrogacy is seen by some as a bioethical issue.

_____

_____

_____

_____

_____

© 2015 Pearson Education, Inc.

CHAPTER 6
Interpersonal Communication Skills

CHAPTER OUTLINE

COMPETENCY SKILLS PERFORMANCE

CHAPTER REVIEW

- Communication is the process of sharing ideas between two or more people. It is the transfer of information and can take different forms, such as sending messages verbally and nonverbally.

- Communication skills are vital for anyone working in health care, including the medical assistant.

- The medical assistant must have a firm understanding of the communication process in order to share information accurately with patients, physicians, and coworkers, and to respond appropriately.

- The communication process includes a source, message, channel, receiver, and feedback.

© 2015 Pearson Education, Inc.

- The medical assistant must use various tools and techniques to overcome communication barriers, such as with patients who do not speak English as their primary language, or patients with special needs, such as those who are deaf, or patients who have a speech impediment that makes them difficult to understand.
- An important part of proper communication is knowing when the use of therapeutic touch and therapeutic communication are appropriate.
- Other challenges to communicating in the medical office include working with angry or distressed patients and working with children.
- The medical assistant must be aware of the various referral resources that the physician may recommend for the patient. These resources include a variety of support groups or other places where patients may seek help for their particular needs.
- Because patient safety is of utmost importance, all members of the health care team must be able to communicate with each other in a clear manner while maintaining patient confidentiality. The medical assistant must also effectively communicate with other health care facilities.
- The medical assistant is responsible for educating patients regarding new skills or in the use of medical equipment. Patient education consists of supplying information about the patient's condition and treatment options and supplying the patient with resources where he or she might seek further information.
- Medical assistants must be aware of the various communication challenges that may arise when educating patients.

LEARNING ACTIVITIES

To ensure that you have achieved the learning objectives in this chapter:

1. In the Terminology Review section on page 51, define the key terminology found in this chapter of your student text.

2. Describe a situation in communicating with a patient that describes both verbal and nonverbal communication, including how each can be used most effectively.

_____
_____
_____
_____
_____

3. Review the different types of listening skills described in this chapter. Which of these listening skills do you feel you excel at? What can you do to improve the skills that don't come as naturally to you?

_____
_____
_____
_____
_____

4. Describe a situation with a patient where you might encounter a communication barrier. Describe how you would overcome this barrier.

_____
_____

© 2015 Pearson Education, Inc.

_____

_____

_____

5. Imagine you are communicating with an angry patient. Describe how you would handle this situation.

_____

_____

_____

_____

_____

6. Imagine you are communicating with a difficult patient. Describe how you would handle this situation.

_____

_____

_____

_____

_____

7. Think of a culture other than your own. Describe the culture, then describe how you would communicate effectively with a patient from this culture.

_____

_____

_____

_____

_____

APPLIED LEARNING EXERCISES

Using a separate sheet of paper, complete the following assignments:

1. Create a list of the various community resources in your area that may be used for patient referrals.
2. Write an essay that outlines the ways to communicate effectively with other members of the health care team.
3. Design patient education material that could be used to educate a patient in the ambulatory care setting.

TERMINOLOGY REVIEW

Using the glossary and highlighted terms in the textbook, define the following terms:

active listening: _____

_____

assess: _____

_____

body language: _____

_____

close-ended question: _____

_____

discriminating: _____

_____

documenting: _____

_____

empathy: _____

_____

evaluation: _____

_____

examples: _____

_____

feedback: _____

_____

implementation: _____

_____

open-ended question: _____

_____

personal space: _____

_____

planning: _____

_____

professional distance: _____

_____

reflecting: _____

_____

stereotyping: _____

_____

sympathy: _____

_____

therapeutic communication: _____

_____

CRITICAL THINKING QUESTIONS

1. Miles O'Brien, CMA (AAMA), is working in a cardiology practice. The physician has asked Miles to use the Internet to locate information for a patient education pamphlet that describes dietary changes that can be made to reduce high cholesterol. How should Miles proceed with this task?

_____

_____

© 2015 Pearson Education, Inc.

_____
_____
_____
_____

2. Gloria Quark, RMA (AMT), is working in a family practice clinic. Her patient is Thomas Nelson, a 55-year-old man who has recently been diagnosed with high cholesterol, high blood pressure, and obesity. Mr. Nelson's physician wants Gloria to give Mr. Nelson information on how to change his diet to lose weight and bring down his blood pressure and cholesterol level. How should Gloria begin this project? What factors about the patient's lifestyle should she consider?

_____
_____
_____
_____
_____

3. Benjamin Shipley, CMA (AAMA), is working with Ms. Marian Harrison, a 60-year-old patient. Her physician has prescribed a medication that she has never taken before. The physician has asked Benjamin to create a medication teaching tool. What should Benjamin include in this tool?

_____
_____
_____
_____
_____

4. Mark Jensen is a student in a medical assisting program. He has been given an assignment to create an educational sheet for tips to prevent childhood injuries. What sort of information should Mark include?

_____
_____
_____
_____

5. Krystle Guthmiller, NCMA (NCCT), is working in a busy internal medicine clinic. Her patient is Ms. Vicky Wagner, an 85-year-old woman with severe arthritis in her hands. The physician has prescribed several medications for Ms. Wagner. What sort of considerations should Krystle keep in mind with this patient that may interfere with her ability to open the medication bottles?

_____
_____
_____
_____
_____

CHAPTER REVIEW TEST

MULTIPLE CHOICE

Circle the letter of the correct answer.

1. Which of the following is NOT one of the five Cs of better communication?
   a. Content
   b. Clarity
   c. Coherence
   d. Check
   e. Caution

2. The communication process includes all of the following EXCEPT _____.
   a. the source
   b. the message
   c. the channel
   d. the receiver
   e. the documentation

3. The _____ step of patient education involves checking to see how well patients are using the information given to them.
   a. evaluation
   b. documenting
   c. implementing
   d. planning
   e. assessing

4. The _____ step of patient education is the actual teaching phase.
   a. evaluation
   b. documenting
   c. implementing
   d. planning
   e. assessing

5. The _____ step of patient education includes taking the information gathered during the assessment and determining how to proceed to educate the patient.
   a. evaluation
   b. documenting
   c. implementing
   d. planning
   e. assessing

6. What information should the medical assistant have on hand before calling another facility to schedule a patient referral?
   a. The patient's name and contact information
   b. The reason for the referral
   c. The name of the referring physician
   d. The correct patient file
   e. All of the above

7. Which of the following is the proper way to address a physician named Mark Winsome, MD, in front of patients?
   a. Dr. Mark
   b. Mark
   c. Dr. Winsome
   d. Physician Mark
   e. None of the above

© 2015 Pearson Education, Inc.

8. Which of the following conversations between coworkers in the medical office would be considered inappropriate if done within patient hearing range?

   a. A discussion of the status of an order of office supplies

   b. A discussion of an upcoming educational seminar on the use of a new piece of office equipment

   c. A discussion of the plot from a television show from the night before

   d. A discussion of the physician's travel plans to an upcoming conference

   e. None of the above

9. Which of the following is an example of NOT keeping a professional distance between the medical assistant and the patient?

   a. The medical assistant offering to give the patient a ride home from the clinic

   b. The medical assistant giving the patient educational materials about smoking cessation

   c. The medical assistant listening to the patient describe her wedding plans

   d. The medical assistant going out to lunch with a coworker

   e. None of the above

10. In order to be HIPAA compliant, how should the medical assistant call a patient named Carol Wisowski from the reception room?

    a. Carol Wisowski

    b. Carol

    c. Ms. Carol Wisowski

    d. Ms. W

    e. Any of the above

TRUE/FALSE

Identify whether the statement is true (T) or false (F).

_____ 1. The medical assistant should never use pet names for patients, such as "sweetie" or "hon."

_____ 2. In order to maintain HIPAA compliance, the medical assistant should refer to the patient as a medical condition, rather than by name.

_____ 3. Medical assistants should never shorten a patient's name without the patient's consent to do so.

_____ 4. There is a "right" way to grieve.

_____ 5. When working with a patient who is grieving a loss, it is appropriate for the medical assistant to share his or her own losses with the patient.

_____ 6. When working with teenagers, the medical assistant should direct the conversation solely to the parent, since the patient is a minor.

_____ 7. If a patient becomes upset, the proper response is for the medical assistant to leave the room.

_____ 8. When working with a patient who has an interpreter, the medical assistant should direct all conversation to the interpreter, not to the patient.

_____ 9. When working with a patient who has a speech impediment that makes his spoken word difficult to understand, it is appropriate for the medical assistant to ask the patient to write down his answers.

_____ 10. When working with a sight-impaired patient, the medical assistant should familiarize the patient with the treatment room's layout and important features, such as the sink and the door.

SHORT ANSWER

1. Explain how the medical assistant should work with a patient who brings a service animal, such as a seeing-eye dog, to the appointment.

   _____

   _____

   _____

   _____

2. What are some tips for working with a hearing-impaired patient?

   _____

   _____

   _____

   _____

3. Define stereotyping and discriminating. What is the difference between the two?

   _____

   _____

   _____

   _____

4. Explain the difference between direct and indirect questions. Give an example of each.

   _____

   _____

   _____

   _____

   _____

5. What is the purpose for allowing periods of silence in conversations with patients?

   _____

   _____

   _____

   _____

   _____

6. What are the basic human needs according to Maslow?

   _____

   _____

   _____

   _____

   _____

© 2015 Pearson Education, Inc.

7. How does the medical assistant demonstrate active listening with the patient?

_____

_____

_____

_____

_____

8. What is meant by "personal space"?

_____

_____

_____

_____

_____

9. What are the five stages of grief according to Dr. Elisabeth Kübler-Ross?

_____

_____

_____

_____

_____

10. Describe the use of therapeutic communication with patients. What techniques are used, and how can they improve the communication process?

_____

_____

_____

_____

_____

CHAPTER 7
Written Communication

CHAPTER OUTLINE

COMPETENCY SKILLS PERFORMANCE

CHAPTER REVIEW

- Written documents are sent from the medical office on a regular basis. Physicians will send letters to patients, to other physicians, or to business associates. Since the administrative medical assistant is often called upon to compose these letters for the physician, a thorough understanding of how to compose a professional business letter is extremely important.

- From the use of proper grammar to correct spelling and punctuation, any letter that is sent from the medical office is a reflection of the professionalism of the entire office and therefore must be both professional and accurate. Due to the potential for miscommunication and possible patient injury if mistakes are made when writing a letter regarding patient care or diagnosis, accuracy is crucial.

© 2015 Pearson Education, Inc.

- The proofreading of business letters, which involves attention to detail as well as a solid understanding of English essentials, is a means by which the medical assistant can help support a positive professional image for the office.
- Abbreviations are common in medical terminology. For all members of the health care team, however, it is essential to use only accepted abbreviations in office communication. The Joint Commission (TJC) has identified the standard abbreviations its members are required to use, as well as avoid.
- Memos are commonly used in the medical office to provide communication between two or more staff members.
- The administrative medical assistant will often be responsible for mailing written letters from the medical office. This task requires an understanding of the rules and restrictions of the U.S. mail system, how to use security or window envelopes, and how to determine the proper postage for a particular item.
- E-mail is another form of written communication used in the medical office. It is governed by its own unique set of rules and policies. The medical assistant must be able to determine how to use this communication technique while maintaining patient confidentiality.
- The administrative medical assistant is commonly assigned the task of opening and distributing the mail within the medical office, as well as annotating the physician's correspondence.

LEARNING ACTIVITIES

To ensure that you have achieved the learning objectives in this chapter:

1. In the Terminology Review section on page 60, define the key terminology found in this chapter of your student text.
2. Go to the USPS Web site. Describe how mail is classified.

_____

_____

_____

_____

_____

_____

APPLIED LEARNING EXERCISES

Using a separate sheet of paper, complete the following assignments:

1. Write a brief essay that outlines how correct grammar, spelling, and punctuation are used in professional communication.
2. Compose a letter to a new patient welcoming the patient to the practice.
3. Write a brief essay that details the process of proofreading a business letter.
4. Using the Internet as a research source, create a list of accepted health care abbreviations.
5. Create a sample memo that might be sent in the medical office.
6. Write an office policy that outlines how an office might handle incoming and outgoing e-mails to patients.
7. Write an office policy that describes how incoming mail and correspondence might be handled in a medical office.

TERMINOLOGY REVIEW

Using the glossary and highlighted terms in the textbook, define the following terms:

annotation: _____

_____

body: _____

_____

closing: _____

_____

electronic mail: _____

_____

font: _____

_____

letterhead: _____

_____

logo: _____

_____

memo: _____

_____

postage meter: _____

_____

proofreader's marks: _____

_____

proofreading: _____

_____

reference initials: _____

_____

salutation: _____

_____

spell check: _____

_____

subject line: _____

_____

thesaurus: _____

_____

ABBREVIATIONS

Provide the meanings of the following abbreviations:

ECG: _____

JCAHO: _____

© 2015 Pearson Education, Inc.

MLOCR: _____

OCR: _____

PDR: _____

TJC: _____

UPS: _____

USPS: _____

CRITICAL THINKING QUESTIONS

1. Missie Hurst, RMA (AMT), is working as an administrative medical assistant with a gastroenterology practice. Dr. Brown has asked Missie to annotate the laboratory reports that come back from the lab. What is he asking Missie to do?

_____

_____

_____

_____

_____

_____

2. Henry Connelly, CMAA (NHA), has just been hired to work at the front desk in a family practice clinic. Part of his job is to open and sort the mail. There is no written office policy about this task currently on file in the office so Henry decides to create one. How should Henry proceed, and what might his policy look like?

_____

_____

_____

_____

_____

3. Willie Rachenko, RMA (AMT), has been working with Dr. Stuart for several years. Dr. Stuart asks Willie to contact Mr. Brocheer with his lab results from earlier this week. Willie looks into Mr. Brocheer's chart and sees that the patient has listed his work e-mail address. Willie isn't able to reach Mr. Brocheer by telephone and instead of leaving a voicemail message asking the patient to return his call, Willie decides to e-mail the patient with his lab results. Later that day, Mr. Brocheer calls the office, very upset. He tells Willie that his boss intercepted the e-mail and now knows that his employee was screened for a sexually transmitted infection. What did Willie do wrong?

_____

_____

_____

_____

_____

_____

© 2015 Pearson Education, Inc.

4. Mallory Valdez is taking an administrative medical assisting class. She has been given the assignment of writing a short paper that outlines the various mailing services offered by the U.S. Postal Service. What should Mallory include in her paper?

_____

_____

_____

_____

_____

5. Ronna Howard, CMA (AAMA), is an administrative medical assistant at the Valley View Clinic. She received an e-mail from a patient, Mrs. Margaret Banks, requesting the results of her laboratory work. How should Ronna respond to this patient?

_____

_____

_____

_____

_____

CHAPTER REVIEW TEST

MULTIPLE CHOICE

Circle the letter of the correct answer.

1. Which of the following organizations has identified the standard abbreviations its members are required to use, as well as avoid?
   a. Occupational Safety and Health Administration (OSHA)
   b. United Parcel Service (UPS)
   c. U.S. Food and Drug Administration (FDA)
   d. The Joint Commission (TJC)
   e. Drug Enforcement Agency (DEA)

2. Which of the following is the size of a standard business envelope?
   a. $3^{1}/_{2}'' \times 8^{1}/_{2}''$
   b. $4^{1}/_{8}'' \times 9^{1}/_{2}''$
   c. $4^{1}/_{4}'' \times 9^{1}/_{4}''$
   d. $8^{1}/_{2}'' \times 11''$
   e. None of the above

3. _____ is used strictly for printed or bound materials, such as books or magazines, videotapes, or DVDs.
   a. Certified mail
   b. First-class mail
   c. Express mail
   d. Priority mail
   e. Media Mail

© 2015 Pearson Education, Inc.

4. Which of the following services should the administrative medical assistant use to mail an item that must arrive by the next day?
   a. Express mail
   b. Priority mail
   c. Media Mail
   d. First-class mail
   e. Priority mail flat rate

5. The _____ is the USPS system of using five digits to indicate mail's intended destination.
   a. multiline optical character reader
   b. optical character recognition
   c. area code
   d. zip code
   e. None of the above

6. Martin F. Susman, MD, has dictated a letter to a patient. The medical assistant who types the letter is Kendra M. Oncler, CMA (AAMA). Which of the following is the correct way to use the reference initials on the letter?
   a. MS/KO
   b. MFS/KMO
   c. ms/ko
   d. MFS/kmo
   e. KMO/MFS

7. The _____ of a professional letter typically appears two lines down from the ending portion of the body.
   a. closing
   b. subject line
   c. salutation
   d. letterhead
   e. body

8. Which of the following pieces of information is typically included in the office letterhead?
   a. The office name
   b. The office address
   c. The office e-mail address
   d. The office telephone and fax number
   e. All of the above

9. Which of the following statements is written correctly?
   a. The patient is taking five milligrams of the medication every hour.
   b. The patient is taking 5 milligrams of the medication every hour.
   c. The patient is taking five (5) milligrams of the medication every hour.
   d. All of the above are correct.
   e. None of the above are correct.

10. Which of the following words is misspelled?
   a. Foriegn
   b. Occurrence
   c. Liaison
   d. Accidentally
   e. Believe

TRUE/FALSE

Identify whether the statement is true (T) or false (F).

_____ 1. If the medical assistant is unsure of the proper spelling of a medical term, she should look the word up in a medical dictionary.

_____ 2. Any word-processing program will accurately spell check medical terms.

_____ 3. Many medical offices maintain social media sites as a form of marketing and advertising to the community.

_____ 4. A professional letter to a patient should address one topic per paragraph.

_____ 5. Physicians will frequently provide just basic facts and ask their medical assistant to compose letters with more detail.

_____ 6. Many medical offices send text messages to patients as reminders of their appointments.

_____ 7. Mail marked "Personal" or "Confidential" should be opened by the medical assistant, then placed on the physician's desk.

_____ 8. Since mail sent to the medical office may contain private patient information, it should never be left where other people can access it, even if it is unopened.

_____ 9. Because confidentiality is not guaranteed, medical staff should use e-mail only to send nonconfidential information.

_____ 10. "Ms." is used when a woman's marital status is unknown, or when the woman prefers.

SHORT ANSWER

1. What are the restricted items mentioned in this chapter that cannot be sent via the USPS?

_____

_____

_____

_____

_____

2. How are multiline optical character readers used in the postal system?

_____

_____

_____

_____

_____

3. What are the restrictions for using Media Mail or standard mail with the USPS?

_____

_____

_____

_____

_____

4. How are memos typically used in the medical office?

_____

_____

_____

_____

_____

5. List the medical abbreviations to avoid that are described in this chapter and list the potential problem with using these abbreviations.

_____

_____

© 2015 Pearson Education, Inc.

_____

_____

_____

6. What are the benefits to having a list of accepted medical abbreviations available for all staff members in the medical office?

_____

_____

_____

_____

7. Describe the process of proofreading.

_____

_____

_____

_____

8. Describe two reasons why the medical office might send a letter to one of its patients.

_____

_____

_____

_____

9. Define the following business letter formats: block format, modified block format, and modified block with indentations.

_____

_____

_____

10. Write an office policy for how an office might handle a situation where the physician will be out of the office when letters must be mailed.

_____

_____

_____

_____

© 2015 Pearson Education, Inc.

CHAPTER 8
Telephone Procedures

CHAPTER OUTLINE

COMPETENCY SKILLS PERFORMANCE

CHAPTER REVIEW

- Professional, proper use of the telephone is essential for the medical assistant. Since the telephone is often the patient's first contact with the medical office, the telephone call is extremely important in making a good first impression.

- The medical assistant must be familiar with the features available on the office telephone system and be able to use those features as needed for added job convenience.

- Many medical offices use answering services when the office is closed or the receptionist or administrative medical assistant is unavailable.

- Since most medical offices have multiple telephone lines that come into the office, the medical assistant must be able to prioritize the callers in an appropriate manner. The process of answering multiple telephone lines includes properly triaging telephone calls and handling possible emergencies on the telephone.

- To triage the medical office's incoming calls properly, medical assistants need a distinct skill set, including a good understanding of any procedure's time requirements.

© 2015 Pearson Education, Inc.

- Emergency calls dictate special telephone attention, as do callers who are angry or otherwise upset.
- Some offices incorporate the use of a patient telephone in the medical office. These telephones are typically located in a patient area of the office, such as the reception room, and are available for the patients to use.
- The administrative medical assistant's duties may include screening incoming telephone calls. This task includes gathering information from the caller, then determining if the call should be put through to the physician or if a message should be taken.
- When taking telephone messages in the office, the administrative medical assistant must be sure to gather all necessary information as well as be certain names are spelled correctly and numbers are written as given. When patients call and give relevant medical information to the medical assistant, the call must be documented accurately in the patient's chart.
- Telephone directories, both electronic and conventional hard-copy versions, are helpful tools in the office's search for telephone numbers. Prescription requests must be made using proper, professional telephone procedure.
- Medical assistants must be careful to maintain patient confidentiality when using the office telephone.

LEARNING ACTIVITIES

To ensure that you have achieved the learning objectives in this chapter:

1. In the Terminology Review section on page 68, define the key terminology found in this chapter of your student text.

2. List and describe five features of a multifeature telephone system.

_____

_____

_____

_____

_____

_____

3. Create a list that describes the benefits of using an answering service in the medical office.

_____

_____

_____

_____

_____

4. Describe the proper procedure for taking an emergency telephone call in the medical office when the patient needs immediate transport to the hospital.

_____

_____

_____

_____

_____

5. Create a list of suggestions for using a telephone directory effectively.

_____

_____

6. Match the caller with the person the call should be transferred to:
   a. Potential call recipients: The physician, the office manager, the receptionist, the clinical medical assistant, the registered nurse
   b. Callers: A pharmaceutical representative with information on a new medication, a medical assistant calling about the possibility of employment in the office, a local pharmacist with a request for a prescription refill, a new patient seeking information about services in the office

APPLIED LEARNING EXERCISES

Using a separate sheet of paper, complete the following assignments:

1. Create a step-by-step procedure for performing telephone triage.
2. Create a step-by-step procedure for taking a proper telephone message.
3. Create a step-by-step procedure for responding to telephone prescription requests.
4. Write a brief essay that discusses how the medical assistant can protect patient confidentiality while using the telephone.

TERMINOLOGY REVIEW

Using the glossary and highlighted terms in the textbook, define the following terms:

automatic dialer: _____

_____

automatic routing unit: _____

_____

call forwarding: _____

_____

conference call: _____

_____

direct telephone lines: _____

_____

established patient: _____

_____

generic message: _____

_____

hands-free telephone device: _____

_____

hold feature: _____

_____

last number redial: _____

_____

© 2015 Pearson Education, Inc.

route: _____

speaker phone: _____

_____

speed dial: _____

_____

triage notebook: _____

_____

triaging: _____

_____

Web chat: _____

_____

ABBREVIATIONS

Provide the meanings of the following abbreviations:

ADA: _____

HIPAA: _____

TTY: _____

CRITICAL THINKING QUESTIONS

1. Rosie Sanchez, CMA (AAMA), has been working as an administrative medical assistant in an internal medicine clinic for the past year. A large part of her day is spent answering the office telephone and scheduling appointments. She would like the office to provide her with a hands-free headset for the telephone system. The clinic director has asked Rosie to create a list that outlines the benefits of having a hands-free headset over a conventional telephone headset. What should Rosie list?

   _____

   _____

   _____

   _____

   _____

2. Mackenzie Quinn, RMA (AMT), has just been hired to work as an administrative medical assistant in a family practice clinic. While checking in a new patient at the front desk, Mackenzie's cell phone rings. She puts a finger up to the patient, to indicate she will need a moment, and then answers the call. The medical office manager witnesses Mackenzie having a conversation on her cell phone regarding her dinner plans that evening. What might the medical office manager say to Mackenzie regarding personal cell phone use in the medical office?

   _____

   _____

   _____

3. Ron Douglas, RMA (AMT), is the front desk receptionist at a busy family medical practice. When Ron answers the phone, he is greeted by an irate patient who is yelling and complaining that she still has not received the results of her lab work. How should Ron handle this patient?

_____

_____

_____

_____

_____

4. Yelena Sheytovski, CMAS (AMT), is working with Dr. Francis. The office has just purchased a new telephone system that allows the user to record telephone calls. Dr. Francis has asked Yelena to create a recorded message to alert callers that their call may be recorded. What should Yelena's message include?

_____

_____

_____

_____

_____

5. Martin Taylor, RMA (AMT), is working in an audiology clinic. The clinic is researching the possibility of purchasing a new telephone system that will include an automatic routing unit where callers can dial an extension to reach their desired party. Martin has been asked to create a list of pros and cons for this type of system. What should Martin include on his list?

_____

_____

_____

_____

_____

CHAPTER REVIEW TEST

MULTIPLE CHOICE

Circle the letter of the correct answer.

1. Which of the following would be appropriate to play for callers who are on hold?
   a. A local radio station
   b. Prerecorded music
   c. A message about seasonal allergies
   d. A message about an upcoming flu shot clinic
   e. All of the above

                    © 2015 Pearson Education, Inc.

2. Which of the following might be offensive or irritating for callers to listen to while they are on hold?

   a. Religious music
   b. Prerecorded music
   c. A message about seasonal allergies
   d. A local radio station
   e. A message about an upcoming flu shot clinic

3. How long is an acceptable period of time to leave a caller on hold?

   a. Less than 10 seconds
   b. 20–30 seconds
   c. 45–60 seconds
   d. 1–2 minutes
   e. 2–3 minutes

4. Generally, offices require at least _____ hours' notice to refill prescriptions.

   a. 2
   b. 12
   c. 24
   d. 36
   e. 48

5. The medical office telephone should be answered _____.

   a. on the first ring
   b. within 2–3 rings
   c. within 3–4 rings
   d. on the fifth ring
   e. None of the above

6. Which of the following pieces of information should the medical assistant be prepared to give callers?

   a. Directions to the office
   b. Parking fees
   c. Parking availability
   d. The insurance plans the physician is participating with
   e. All of the above

7. Which of the following telephone calls should be taken care of first?

   a. A patient who says she needs to schedule her yearly mammogram
   b. An angry patient who is calling about her bill
   c. A patient who says he is having chest pain
   d. A patient who is calling to find out his laboratory results
   e. A patient who is calling for directions to the office

8. What information would you expect to find in a telephone triage notebook?

   a. Driving directions to the medical office
   b. The hours the clinic is open
   c. The types of insurance accepted at the medical office
   d. The questions to ask a patient who complains of chest pain
   e. All of the above

9. In the event of a medical emergency in the office, what information should the medical assistant have available before calling for emergency services?

   a. The patient's name
   b. The patient's age
   c. The patient's gender
   d. The problem type
   e. All of the above

10. Which of the following types of patient calls would NOT typically require charting?

    a. Patients who cancel appointments and fail to reschedule
    b. Patients who say they are in the hospital
    c. Patients who indicate they are not returning to the office for care
    d. Patients who indicate they cannot afford to keep their appointments
    e. Patients confirming appointment times

TRUE/FALSE

Identify whether the statement is true (T) or false (F).

_____ 1. The medical assistant should always ask a caller for permission before placing the caller on hold.

_____ 2. When choosing a staff member to record a message for the office telephone hold feature, the person with the most pleasant voice should make the recording.

_____ 3. In order to give patients the highest quality of customer service, medical offices should use answering services that are experienced in health care.

_____ 4. Medical assistants should have coworkers' cell phone numbers available to give to callers in the event the coworker is not in the office when the caller calls.

_____ 5. The medical assistant should attempt to match the caller's rate of speech when talking on the telephone.

_____ 6. In general, it is most efficient to address short telephone calls before longer ones.

_____ 7. The medical assistant should never chew gum while answering the office telephone.

_____ 8. In the event an upset or angry patient calls the office, the medical assistant should place the caller on hold to give him or her time to calm down.

_____ 9. Most medical offices require at least 72 hours' notice to refill prescriptions.

_____ 10. The medical assistant should consider time zones when making long distance telephone calls.

SHORT ANSWER

1. What should a medical office consider before choosing a type of music to use for the on hold feature?

_____

_____

_____

_____

_____

2. Explain how automatic redial in reverse works.

_____

_____

_____

_____

_____

3. Explain how telephone triage works.

_____

_____

_____

© 2015 Pearson Education, Inc.

4. Create a list of types of calls from patients that would need to be documented in the patient's chart.

_____

_____

_____

_____

_____

5. What items must be written down when taking a telephone message?

_____

_____

_____

_____

_____

6. Write an office policy for leaving telephone messages on a patient's voicemail.

_____

_____

_____

_____

_____

7. What information would the medical assistant need to give another health care facility when calling to schedule a patient for an appointment?

_____

_____

_____

_____

_____

8. What are some telephone tips the medical assistant can use to show patients courtesy?

_____

_____

_____

_____

9. Write an office policy on how a medical office might regulate the use of the office telephone for personal telephone calls.

_____

_____

_____

_____

_____

10. Describe how a telephone telecommunication relay service works.

_____

_____

_____

_____

_____

© 2015 Pearson Education, Inc.

CHAPTER 9
Front Desk Reception

CHAPTER OUTLINE

COMPETENCY SKILLS PERFORMANCE

CHAPTER REVIEW

- The front desk receptionist is the host or hostess in the medical clinic. The receptionist is typically the first person the patient will speak with on the telephone when making an appointment and the first face the patient will see upon arriving at the medical office.

- The reception area in a medical office should be decorated in a manner that suits the type of patients who will seek treatment there. Reception rooms should always be safe and clean and should have an attractive, welcoming, and calm environment for patients as they wait their turn to see the physician.

- The medical office receptionist should exhibit certain personality traits. These include friendliness, compassion, extreme attention to detail, and the ability to handle many tasks at once.

© 2015 Pearson Education, Inc.

- The receptionist is typically the person who will open the office at the beginning of the day, preparing patient charts and other items as necessary in order to be ready for patient arrivals. At the end of the day, it is the receptionist who will typically close the office, finishing any uncompleted work from the day and preparing items for the next morning.

- Throughout the day, the receptionist will typically be responsible for keeping an eye on the reception area, making sure that any garbage is picked up and that the room remains safe from items or furniture that may have been moved and might cause a safety concern.

- The receptionist must keep the patients in the reception room abreast of any delays or changes in the schedule that may cause the patient to wait longer than expected. By alerting patients to these delays right away, the medical receptionist can keep a patient from getting angry over the lack of communication.

- The medical receptionist is often stationed adjacent to the reception area; therefore, any conversations that go on between the receptionist and the patient might be overheard by other patients who are waiting to see the physician. The medical receptionist must maintain patient privacy and be aware of when a conversation should be moved to another area of the office.

LEARNING ACTIVITIES

To ensure that you have achieved the learning objectives in this chapter:

1. In the Terminology Review section on page 78, define the key terminology found in this chapter of your student text.

2. Create a list of the steps to opening the medical office.

_____

_____

_____

_____

_____

_____

_____

_____

_____

_____

3. Imagine you are working at the front desk in a medical clinic. A new patient calls the office and refuses to give the reason for his need to see the physician. Create a list of suggestions for persuading this patient to provide the needed information.

_____

_____

_____

_____

_____

_____

4. Imagine you are working at the front desk in a medical clinic. One of your physicians has just called to say she is going to be an hour late coming to the office. You already have three patients in the reception room waiting to see this physician. Create a list of how you will communicate with these

© 2015 Pearson Education, Inc.

patients, as well as the patients who are scheduled to see this physician for the remainder of the day, regarding the delay.

_____

_____

_____

_____

_____

_____

5. You have the following patients in the reception area: a man with obvious symptoms of the flu, a child with chicken pox blisters, a woman with a sinus infection, a child with conjunctivitis, a teenager who is vomiting into a bag. Outline how you will deal with each of these patients.

_____

_____

_____

_____

_____

_____

_____

6. Create a list of suggestions for maintaining a safe and pleasant reception room environment.

_____

_____

_____

_____

_____

_____

7. Create a list of suggestions for creating a safe children's area in the reception room.

_____

_____

_____

_____

_____

_____

APPLIED LEARNING EXERCISES

Using a separate sheet of paper, complete the following assignments:

1. List the steps the receptionist should take to prepare files for patient arrivals.
2. Write a brief essay that outlines the appropriate ways to greet and register both new and established patients.

3. Create an office policy that identifies means of maintaining patient confidentiality in all front desk activities.

4. Write a brief essay that describes how you would manage a loud and difficult patient who is using abusive language in the reception area.

5. Write a brief essay describing how a medical assistant can be effective at collecting copayments at the front desk.

TERMINOLOGY REVIEW

Using the glossary and highlighted terms in the textbook, define the following terms:

Americans with Disabilities Act (ADA): _____

_____

checklist: _____

_____

copayment: _____

_____

front desk: _____

_____

hazard: _____

_____

HIPAA compliant: _____

_____

office policy: _____

_____

reception area: _____

_____

receptionist: _____

_____

service animal: _____

_____

sign-in sheet: _____

_____

ABBREVIATIONS

Provide the meanings of the following abbreviations:

ADA: _____

HIPAA: _____

© 2015 Pearson Education, Inc.

CRITICAL THINKING QUESTIONS

1. Marcus Winston, RMA (AMT), is the administrative medical assistant at the Queensview Medical Practice. A new patient, Miss Elaina Sills, is hearing impaired and has arrived with an escort. What should Marcus keep in mind when communicating with Miss Sills?

_____

_____

_____

_____

_____

2. Sara Womack, CMA (AAMA), is the medical office manager in a women's health clinic. She has two employees who share the job of front desk receptionist. Aaron Shelley, CMA (AAMA), doesn't like to work at the front desk. He is often short with the patients, some of whom have complained to the physician. Michael Sulley, RMA (AMT), is the other front desk receptionist. Michael has a sunny personality and thoroughly enjoys the fast pace at the front desk. Would the office manager be better serving the patients of the clinic if she moved Aaron out of that position and had Michael work there full-time? Why or why not? What sort of ramifications might occur if the office manager leaves Aaron in the front desk position?

_____

_____

_____

_____

_____

3. Marjorie Sorensen, CMAA (NHA), has just been hired to work as the office manager for Dr. Rodriguez. The doctor tells Marjorie that she has noticed that many tasks are being skipped by the front desk staff when opening the office in the morning. Dr. Rodriguez believes the front desk staff is forgetting these tasks and has asked Marjorie to come up with a solution to this problem. What might Marjorie suggest?

_____

_____

_____

_____

4. Isaiah Chung is taking an administrative medical assisting course as part of his training to become a medical assistant. His instructor has assigned the task of creating an office policy for opening the medical office. How might Isaiah's policy read?

_____

_____

_____

_____

_____

5. Wally Harrison, NCMA (NCCT), has just come back from an administrative medical assisting continuing education workshop. He has learned that many medical offices are sending new patient paperwork to patients in the mail prior to their appointment. How can Wally explain the benefits of doing this to his coworkers and the physicians where he works?

_____

_____

_____

_____

_____

_____

CHAPTER REVIEW TEST

MULTIPLE CHOICE

Circle the letter of the correct answer.

1. If the medical assistant is on the telephone when a patient arrives at the office, what should she do to let the patient know she is aware of the patient's presence?
   a. Make eye contact with the patient, smile, and hold up an index finger to indicate she'll be with the patient in just a moment.
   b. Continue looking down at the desk so that the patient realizes she is on the telephone and won't be able to help right away.
   c. Turn her back to the patient in order to keep the telephone conversation more private.
   d. Immediately hang up on the caller and provide full attention to the patient.
   e. None of the above

2. To track fees, most offices use preprinted fee slips called _____.
   a. encounter forms
   b. patient registration forms
   c. HIPAA compliance forms
   d. health history forms
   e. fee forms

3. When established patients check in at the front desk, what information should the receptionist confirm with the patient?
   a. Patient's address has not changed since the last visit
   b. Patient's insurance carrier remains the same since the last visit
   c. The type of medications the patient is taking
   d. Patient's telephone number has not changed since the last visit
   e. All of the above

4. A patient's _____ is a predetermined amount of money a patient must pay for each physician's visit.
   a. coinsurance
   b. copayment
   c. deductible
   d. allowed amount
   e. balance

    © 2015 Pearson Education, Inc.

5. Patient registration forms should contain which of the following pieces of information?
   a. The patient's home address
   b. The patient's insurance information
   c. The patient's home phone number
   d. The patient's cell phone number
   e. All of the above

6. To ensure billing processes remain up to date, the patient registration form should be verified
   _____.
   a. weekly
   b. monthly
   c. yearly
   d. at every patient vist but no more than once a month
   e. None of the above

7. How should the receptionist respond when confronted with an angry patient?
   a. Move the patient out of the front desk area.
   b. Ask the patient to sit down in the reception room until she has calmed down.
   c. Walk away from the front desk until the patient calms down.
   d. Ask the patient to lower her voice.
   e. Ask the patient to leave the office.

8. Which of the following patients should be moved out of the reception room as soon as possible?
   a. A patient with HIV
   b. A patient with conjunctivitis
   c. A patient with a fever
   d. A patient with a headache
   e. A patient with a sore throat

9. How should the receptionist handle a patient who brings in food to eat while in the reception room?
   a. The receptionist should ignore it unless the patient is making a mess.
   b. The receptionist should ask the patient to share the food with the other patients in the reception room.
   c. The receptionist should ask the patient to take the food outside to finish eating it.
   d. The receptionist should ask the physician to come out and speak with the patient.
   e. None of the above

10. How much seating should the reception room have for patients?
    a. Enough to accommodate 15 minutes' worth of patients per physician, as well as the patient's friends and relatives
    b. Enough to accommodate 30 minutes' worth of patients per physician, as well as the patient's friends and relatives
    c. Enough to accommodate 1 hour's worth of patients per physician, as well as the patient's friends and relatives
    d. Enough to accommodate 2 hours' worth of patients per physician, as well as the patient's friends and relatives
    e. None of the above

TRUE/FALSE

Identify whether the statement is true (T) or false (F).

_____ 1. When a patient's insurance information has changed, the medical assistant should photocopy both sides of the new insurance card.

_____ 2. When delays occur in the medical office, the receptionist should quickly alert the patients who are waiting.

_____ 3. Part of the front desk receptionist's job is to collect necessary copayments from patients as they arrive.

_____ 4. The medical receptionist may need to ask a child to be quiet if that child is disturbing other patients.

_____ 5. Having educational materials in the reception room is very common in the medical office.

_____ 6. Children must not be left unattended by their parents in the medical office, even for short periods of time.

_____ 7. Service animals, such as seeing-eye dogs, must be allowed to accompany their owner throughout the medical office.

_____ 8. In general, medical office staff should arrive at the office 60 minutes before patients are expected to arrive.

_____ 9. The medical receptionist should greet all patients upon arrival, even when busy with other tasks.

_____ 10. Most medical offices today have a window to separate the receptionist's desk and the reception room.

SHORT ANSWER

1. What are some reasons why a patient may refuse to disclose certain personal information on the history form?

   _____
   _____
   _____
   _____
   _____

2. What is one possible ramification for the patient if he refuses to disclose his birth date to the medical office?

   _____
   _____
   _____
   _____
   _____

3. Explain the pros and cons of using an electronic sign at the front desk to broadcast the physicians' schedules.

   _____
   _____

© 2015 Pearson Education, Inc.

_____

_____

_____

4. When the medical assistant calls for "Joe" from the reception room, two men stand up. How can the medical assistant handle this?

_____

_____

_____

_____

_____

5. Describe the type of décor you would find in a pediatric office. What type of décor would you find in a women's health care practice?

_____

_____

_____

_____

_____

6. Describe the types of reading material you would find in a clinic that treats mainly male patients.

_____

_____

_____

_____

_____

7. Explain how the Americans with Disabilities Act applies to the medical office setting.

_____

_____

_____

_____

_____

8. When greeting new patients, what sort of things should the medical assistant do to orient the new patient to the office environment?

_____

_____

_____

_____

_____

9. What is a benefit to using an electronic sign-in sheet in the medical office?

_____

_____

_____

_____

_____

© 2015 Pearson Education, Inc.

10. If the medical receptionist has a patient arrive who cannot fill out his own paperwork, how can the medical assistant assist this patient?

_____

_____

_____

_____

_____

                                    © 2015 Pearson Education, Inc.

CHAPTER 10
Scheduling

CHAPTER OUTLINE

Introduction
Scheduling New Patient Appointments
Electronic Scheduling
Methods of Appointment Scheduling
Correcting the Appointment Schedule
Documenting No-Show Appointments
Managing the Physician's Professional Schedule
Scheduling Hospital Services and Admissions
Arranging for Language Interpreters
Arranging Transportation for Patients
Achieving Efficiency in Scheduling
Review

COMPETENCY SKILLS PERFORMANCE

Procedure 10-1: Establish an Appointment Matrix
Procedure 10-2: Schedule a New Patient Appointment
Procedure 10-3: Schedule an Established Patient Appointment
Procedure 10-4: Use Patient Reminder Cards
Procedure 10-5: Reschedule a Missed Patient Appointment
Procedure 10-6: Manage the Physician's Professional Schedule and Travel
Procedure 10-7: Schedule a Hospital Procedure
Procedure 10-8: Schedule an Inpatient Admission

CHAPTER REVIEW

- Efficient appointment scheduling is vital to the successful operation of a medical office. The administrative medical assistant who is assigned the task of answering the office telephone must be well versed in how to schedule both new and established patients using different methods of appointment scheduling, as well as how to handle special situations, such as emergencies, patients who are difficult to understand, and emotional patients. Guidelines for scheduling patient appointments are invaluable tools for medical offices intent on providing effective, efficient patient service.

- When a new patient calls the office to schedule a new patient appointment, it is important to collect specific information while remaining professional, objective, and consistent. A new patient checklist can help ensure that the medical assistant asks appropriate questions.

- Many medical offices choose to mail forms to new patients to fill out prior to their first visit; others ask patients to come in 10–20 minutes prior to their appointment to fill out the paperwork in the office. Many medical offices have copies of the forms patients will be required to fill out on the medical office Web site. Patients can be directed to the Web site and asked to download and fill out the forms, bringing those forms in at the time of their visit. In some medical clinics, patients can fill out the forms online, without having to print out or bring in any paper versions.

- Medical offices have varying policies on what constitutes a *new* and an *established* patient. In general, a new patient has not been seen in the medical office by any of the health care providers of the same specialty within the past 3 years. An established patient has seen one of the health care providers of the same specialty in the medical office within the past 3 years.

- Patients should be made aware of the amount of time they can expect to spend in the office, as well as be kept up to date on any changes in the schedule upon arriving in the office.

- Most medical offices have a set period of time that a particular type of patient appointment is expected to take. Typically, new patients are scheduled for more time than established patients. Each medical office should document its policy for allotting appointment time and review it regularly to ensure it continues to be appropriate for patients and physicians.

- Today, most large medical offices use computer software to manage their patient appointments. Computerized systems vary, depending on the specific needs of the medical practice. Electronic appointment scheduling offers many advantages, some of which are speed and efficiency, access to schedules from different locations within the office, and the ability to schedule multiple physicians at the same time, from any computer in the medical office.

- There are still some physician offices that use paper appointment books. Whether paper or electronic, the appointment book is considered a legal document and must be handled in such a way as to safeguard patient privacy.

- Both paper and electronic scheduling systems accommodate patient no-shows, which always must be documented for legal and other purposes.

- Whenever patients miss their appointments, the medical assistant should follow up to attempt rescheduling.

- Many physicians attend professional meetings outside the office. In many offices, the administrative medical assistant is responsible for managing the physician's professional schedule.

- In addition to scheduling patient appointments in the medical office, medical assistants will also need to schedule patients for procedures or admissions in the hospital, both as inpatients and as outpatients.

- Effective medical assistants arrange appropriate transportation services or language interpreters for patients who need them.

LEARNING ACTIVITIES

To ensure that you have achieved the learning objectives in this chapter:

1. In the Terminology Review section on page 88, define the key terminology found in this chapter of your student text.

2. Using the provided appointment book sheet in Figure 10-1, refer to Table 10-1 in your student textbook (Time Allotted for Patient Appointments), and write the following patients into the appointment schedule (be sure to indicate the amount of time each patient will need):
   a. Monica Gypsym, a new patient coming in for a physical exam at 10:00 A.M.
   b. Sydney Crossett, an established patient coming in for a blood pressure check at 11:15 A.M.
   c. Mark Jensen, an established teenage patient coming in for a physical exam at 2:00 P.M.
   d. Anthony Garcia, a new patient coming in for a routine checkup at 9:00 A.M.

3. Using the same appointment book sheet used for activity 2 (Figure 10-1), indicate that Anthony Garcia has called and moved his appointment to 4:00 P.M.

© 2015 Pearson Education, Inc.

		SERV.	COLL.	R/S		SERV.	COLL.	R/S		SERV.	COLL.	R/S		SERV.	COLL.
9															
9^{15}															
9^{30}															
9^{45}															
10															
10^{15}															
10^{30}															
10^{45}															
11															
11^{15}															
11^{30}															
11^{45}															
12^{00}															
12^{15}															
12^{30}															
12^{45}															
1^{00}															
1^{15}															
1^{30}															
1^{45}															
2^{00}															
2^{15}															
2^{30}															
2^{45}															
3^{00}															
3^{15}															
3^{30}															
3^{45}															

Figure 10-1

© 2015 Pearson Education, Inc.

4. List five advantages of electronic appointment scheduling.

_____

_____

_____

_____

_____

_____

APPLIED LEARNING EXERCISES

Using a separate sheet of paper, complete the following assignments:

1. Using the Internet as a research source, search for three companies that offer software for electronic scheduling. Create a list of features that each company offers.
2. Write an office policy for how to follow up on patients who miss their appointments.
3. Create an office policy for managing the physician's appointment calendar for professional travel.
4. Write a step-by-step procedure for how the administrative medical assistant should handle the scheduling of an inpatient procedure.
5. Create an office policy that describes how the administrative medical assistant would arrange for language interpreters for non-English-speaking patients.

TERMINOLOGY REVIEW

Using the glossary and highlighted terms in the textbook, define the following terms:

buffer time: _____

_____

cluster scheduling: _____

_____

double booking: _____

_____

established patient: _____

_____

fixed-appointment scheduling: _____

_____

matrix: _____

_____

modified wave scheduling: _____

_____

new patient: _____

_____

new patient checklist: _____

_____

© 2015 Pearson Education, Inc.

office brochure: _____

open hours: _____

preapprovals: _____

slack time: _____

triage notebook: _____

virtual appointment: _____

wave scheduling: _____

ABBREVIATIONS

Provide the meaning of the following abbreviation:

ECG: _____

CRITICAL THINKING QUESTIONS

1. Dylan Reilly, CMA (AAMA), is working in a busy family practice office. The physicians and staff all agree that the appointment scheduling system is not working, and patients are frequently waiting long periods of time for appointments. How should Dylan go about creating a new scheduling procedure for this office?

   _____

   _____

   _____

   _____

   _____

2. Mallory Shannon, RMA (AMT), works in a busy clinic that uses paper appointment books. The medical office manager has asked Mallory to prepare a list of compelling reasons to switch to electronic scheduling. What key points should Mallory include in her list with regard to the benefits of electronic scheduling?

   _____

   _____

   _____

   _____

   _____

3. Armando Alonso is taking an administrative medical assisting course as part of his medical assisting training. He has been given an assignment to create a list of information that patients should be given in order to help prepare them for medical procedures. What sort of information should Armando list?

_____

_____

_____

_____

_____

4. Anna Simonenko, CMAS (AMT), is working at the front desk in a family practice clinic. Anna has been asked to schedule Roger Edetsberger for a procedure to be performed in the hospital. Anna tells Mr. Edetsberger that she will need to call his insurance company before she can schedule the procedure. He asks, "Why do you need to do that? Can't you just schedule the procedure now and call the insurance company some other time?" How might Anna respond to this patient?

_____

_____

_____

_____

_____

5. Ronna DeLancer, RMA (AMT), is working as an administrative medical assistant for Dr. Angela Chien. Dr. Chien is traveling out of town for a continuing education seminar and has asked Ronna to make all of the arrangements. What sort of arrangements will Ronna likely make for Dr. Chien?

_____

_____

_____

_____

_____

CHAPTER REVIEW TEST

MULTIPLE CHOICE

Circle the letter of the correct answer.

1. How much time should the medical assistant wait before calling a patient who has missed his appointment?

   a. 5–10 minutes   d. 60 minutes
   b. 10–15 minutes   e. 90 minutes
   c. 15–30 minutes

© 2015 Pearson Education, Inc.

2. Which of the following is an acceptable way to note a missed appointment in a paper appointment book?

   a. Use white correction fluid to cover the patient's name.

   b. Use a black marker to obliterate the patient's name.

   c. Use an eraser to remove the patient's name.

   d. Draw a single line through the patient's name.

   e. All of the above

3. Which of the following is a benefit of electronic scheduling systems?

   a. Several staff members can access the appointment schedule at once and from different locations in the office.

   b. Administrative medical assistants have the ability to schedule multiple physicians at the same time, from any computer in the medical office.

   c. Assistants can print out detailed patient information for physicians, such as detailed histories, prior to the patient's visit.

   d. Computer appointment scheduling is faster and easier than paper scheduling for those staff members experienced with the software.

   e. All of the above

4. Which of the following messages would be appropriate to leave on a patient's voicemail?

   a. "This is Martha calling from Dr. Brown's office to remind John of his appointment tomorrow at 9 A.M."

   b. "This is Martha calling from Dr. Brown's office to remind John of his appointment for a culture and sensitivity test tomorrow at 9 A.M."

   c. "This is Martha calling from Dr. Brown's office to remind John of his appointment tomorrow at 9 A.M. You will need to fast for 12 hours prior to this appointment."

   d. "This is Martha calling from Dr. Brown's office to remind John of his appointment tomorrow at 9 A.M. for his flu vaccination."

   e. All of the above

5. A typical reminder card for patient appointments contains which of the following pieces of information?

   a. The date of the upcoming appointment

   b. The time of the upcoming appointment

   c. The name of the medical facility

   d. The medical facility's phone number

   e. All of the above

6. _____ is an appointment scheduling method of leaving certain times of day open to accommodate situations such as patients who call for same-day appointments or physicians who need to catch up on charting.

   a. Buffer time

   b. Cluster scheduling

   c. Double booking

   d. Fixed appointment scheduling

   e. Modified wave scheduling

7. The _____ method of scheduling is where two or three patients are scheduled at the beginning of each hour, followed by single patient appointments every 10–20 minutes for the rest of that hour.

   a. wave

   b. modified wave

   c. open hours

   d. fixed appointment

   e. double booking

8. The _____ method of scheduling is where patients are scheduled only for the first half of each hour. The first patient to arrive is seen first.

    a. wave
    b. modified wave
    c. open hours

    d. fixed appointment
    e. double booking

9. The _____ method of scheduling is most commonly used in walk-in clinics, laboratories, and X-ray facilities where patients are typically seen on a first-come, first-served basis.

    a. wave
    b. modified wave
    c. open hours

    d. fixed appointment
    e. double booking

10. The _____ method of scheduling is one where each patient is given a specific appointment time.

    a. wave
    b. modified wave
    c. open hours

    d. fixed appointment
    e. double booking

TRUE/FALSE

Identify whether the statement is true (T) or false (F).

_____ 1. Many medical offices use automated telephone reminder systems to remind patients of their upcoming appointments.

_____ 2. Cluster scheduling is a system of booking several patients around the same block of time.

_____ 3. The practice type and physician preference determine the appointment scheduling system the medical office will use.

_____ 4. The appointment book is considered a legal document.

_____ 5. Using a paper appointment book over a computerized appointment scheduling system saves time for the medical assistant.

_____ 6. Some computerized appointment systems allow staff and/or physicians to access the appointment schedule from outside the office.

_____ 7. Many physicians prefer to limit certain types of appointments in any given day.

_____ 8. Established patient appointments are typically allotted more time than new patient appointments.

_____ 9. Accidental injury files are often kept separate from the patient's general medical file.

_____ 10. The medical assistant will typically need to ask new patients to come to the office 10–20 minutes early for their first appointment in order to allow time to complete paperwork.

SHORT ANSWER

1. Explain the importance of documenting missed or no-show appointments.

_____

_____

_____

 © 2015 Pearson Education, Inc.

_____

2. What is the purpose of having a triage notebook near the telephone in the medical office?

_____

_____

_____

_____

3. What is a suggestion for handling the scheduling of a patient who is chronically late for appointments?

_____

_____

_____

_____

4. Describe how double booking works in medical office appointment scheduling.

_____

_____

_____

_____

5. Describe how a color-coded system for scheduling appointments in the medical office might be used.

_____

_____

_____

_____

6. Explain why the medical assistant should pay attention to the patient's needs when scheduling patient appointments.

_____

_____

_____

_____

7. When a medical office has a patient who typically requires more than the normally allotted time (due to a disability or complex health issues), how can the medical assistant make other members of the scheduling staff aware of this need?

_____

_____

_____

_____

© 2015 Pearson Education, Inc.

8. Explain how a matrix is used in appointment scheduling.

_____

_____

_____

_____

9. Explain how to differentiate between a "new" and an "established" patient in the medical office.

_____

_____

_____

_____

10. How should the medical assistant respond if a new patient refuses to disclose insurance information when calling to schedule an appointment?

_____

_____

_____

_____

_____

© 2015 Pearson Education, Inc.

CHAPTER 11
Medical Records Management

CHAPTER OUTLINE

COMPETENCY SKILLS PERFORMANCE

CHAPTER REVIEW

- Medical records play an important role in health care delivery, so they must be accurate and complete. Health care providers rely on patients' medical records as accurate depictions of patients. As legal documents, medical records are often the single most important tools health care providers can use to defend against medical malpractice lawsuits. Risk management and quality improvement programs rely on medical records to catch errors in patient care. Insurance companies often request copies of patient medical records to determine the appropriateness of billing codes and reimbursement levels.

- Medical records include four types of patient information: (1) personal information, (2) financial information, (3) medical information, and (4) social information.

- Items sent from other medical facilities will need to be filed within patient charts. These items may include laboratory reports, consultation reports, or X-ray studies.

- The medical care the patient receives must be accurately recorded in order to provide a picture of the care the patient has received from a particular physician or facility.

- There are several different charting styles found in health care, including alphabetic, numeric, and terminal digit. Each facility will mandate the type of charting to be used.

- In order to maintain the highest level of patient safety, the members of the health care team should all use the same medical abbreviations when charting in patient's charts. To that end, a list of accepted abbreviations should be clearly posted for all staff members to view when making entries in a patient's chart.

- Communications with patients, outside of office visits, must be documented in patients' charts when a communication is medically relevant. Such communications include telephone calls or e-mails from patients that relate to those patients' medical care, missed or canceled appointments, or pharmacy requests to refill prescriptions. Each office should have a policy regarding the type of communication that requires charting, and all members of the health care team should closely follow that policy.

- Most medical offices use one of two types of filing systems: (1) alphabetic or (2) numeric. While alphabetic is far more common overall, numeric filing is more common in facilities where patient treatment records must be kept extremely confidential, such as in facilities specializing in mental health, HIV or AIDS treatment, or reproductive health care.

- Cross-referencing is a method of tracking and finding patient files for patients with multiple last names.

- A variety of file storage systems may be found in the medical office. The type used in any specific facility is generally dictated by the needs and storage space available in that facility.

- Patient files fluctuate between active, inactive, and closed status as patients traverse the health care system. Medical records are often separated into different locations, based on whether the file is that of an active patient, an inactive patient, or a closed patient record. Each medical facility will have a definition of each of those categories for medical assistants to follow.

- Knowledge of how and when copies of the patient's medical record may be released is an important part of how HIPAA legislation works to protect patient privacy.

- Any entry made in the patient's medical record must be properly signed by the person who made the entry. No person on the health care team should ever ask another member of the team to make entries for him or her.

- The administrative medical assistant must be aware of the proper and legal way to make corrections in the patient's medical record, as well as the steps to take should the patient ask to make corrections in his or her own medical record.

- Once a paper medical record has been converted into an electronic form, the paper record must be disposed of properly in order to maintain patient confidentiality.

- At times, physicians will participate in medical research and will use their patient files for this purpose. When a patient is on an experimental medication, or participating in any kind of medical research program, that must be carefully documented in the patient's file.

© 2015 Pearson Education, Inc.

LEARNING ACTIVITIES

To ensure that you have achieved the learning objectives in this chapter:

1. In the Terminology Review section on page 99, define the key terminology found in this chapter of your student text.

2. Create a list of steps to take to locate a missing patient file in the medical office.

_____
_____
_____
_____
_____
_____

3. Create a list of reasons why an office would choose to use numeric filing.

_____
_____
_____
_____
_____
_____

4. For the following patients, which would be considered active, inactive, or closed patient files?
   a. Lori Hughes, a patient who has moved out of the state
   b. Quin Tao, a patient who has not been seen in the office for 5 years
   c. Gloria Sanchez, a patient who was in the office for care last week
   d. Sara Womack, a patient who died last year

5. Describe how the medical office can store inactive patient files.

_____
_____
_____
_____
_____

6. Create a list of steps to take to correct an error in a patient's chart.

_____
_____
_____
_____
_____

7. Create a list of steps to take when a patient wishes to make changes to her medical record.

_____
_____

_____

_____

_____

_____

8. Using the operative report in Figure 11-1, annotate the report for the physician using a yellow highlighter pen.

OPERATION DATE: 8/11/xx

PATIENT: ADAM PARCHER

SURGEON: MARIA FERNANDEZ-RAUL, MD

PREOPERATIVE DIAGNOSIS;
Congenital external nasal deformity.

POSTOPERATIVE DIAGNOSIS:
Congenital external nasal deformity.

PROCEDURE:
Aesthetic rhinoplasty

DESCRIPTION OF PROCEDURE:
The patient is a 33-year-old male who presented with concerns for nasal airway obstruction and discontent with the external appearance of his nose. Examination confirms the above-noted concerns with a widened nasal base, palpable and visible dorsal cartilage and nasal bones.

Correction of the external deformity by open rhinoplasty, lowering of the dorsum, lowering of the cartilaginous dorsum, narrowing of the nasal bones, resection and narrowing of the nasal tip, excision of caudal septum and nasal spine were discussed. The nature of the procedures and risks, including bleeding, hematoma, infection, poor wound healing, scarring, asymmetry, airway difficulties, palpable or visible nasal structures and possible need for secondary procedures were all discussed. The patient understands and wishes to proceed as outlined.

FINDINGS:
The patient underwent open rhinoplasty through a columellar chevron incision. The nose was copiously infiltrated with 1% lidocaine with epinephrine prior to incision. The chevron incision was incised and carried to bilateral rim incisions. The nasal skin was then degloved using sharp dissecting scissors. This was opened over the nose up to the root of the nose to allow full exposure. The irregular nasal bones were initially smoothed with a rasp. Excision of the dorsal nasal bone was then carried out using a straight guarded osteotome. Approximately 1 mm thickness of bone was removed. After osteotomy was completed from a low to high position, infracture of the nasal bones was carried out. This provided good narrowing of the nasal base. A small piece of septal cartilage was crushed and flattened using the cartilage crusher and this was placed over the nasal dorsum. Hemostasis was assured. The skin was redraped and closure was carried out using inter-rupted 6-0 Prolene for the columellar and stab incisions. Interrupted 5-0 plain gut sutures were used to close the rim incisions and the septal transfixion incision. Xeroform packs were removed and nasal splints were placed. A second set of Xeroform packs was placed lateral to the nasal splints. The dorsum of the nose was taped and a dorsal thermoplast splint was also placed. The procedure was well tolerated. The posterior throat was suctioned and a throat pack that had been placed at the beginning of the procedure was removed. The patient was awakened and extubated and discharged to the recovery room in stable condition.

Maria Fernandez-Raul, MD

Figure 11-1

© 2015 Pearson Education, Inc.

9. Indicate whether the following information should be listed under S for subjective findings, O for objective findings, A for assessment, or P for plan:
   a. The patient complains of a sore throat. She says she has had these symptoms for 3 days.
   b. The physician believes the patient has strep throat.
   c. The physician has ordered a throat culture and would like the patient to come back in 1 week if symptoms have not subsided.
   d. The patient's blood pressure is 120/78.

APPLIED LEARNING EXERCISES

Using a separate piece of paper, complete the following assignments:

1. Write a brief essay that describes how cross-referencing is used in the medical office.
2. Write an essay that discusses how color coding is used in filing systems.
3. Using the Internet as a research source, research the types of filing systems that may be found in a medical setting. Describe the pros and cons of each system.
4. Write a brief essay that describes the appropriate way to destroy a medical record. Include the reasons why an office may want or need to destroy a medical record.

TERMINOLOGY REVIEW

Using the glossary and highlighted terms in the textbook, define the following terms:

active patient files: _____
_____

advance directives: _____
_____

chief complaint: _____
_____

closed patient files: _____
_____

cross-referencing: _____
_____

electronic health record: _____
_____

electronic signature: _____
_____

financial information: _____
_____

flow charts: _____
_____

inactive patient files: _____
_____

indecipherable: _____
_____

© 2015 Pearson Education, Inc.

medical information: _____

_____

medical record: _____

_____

medical research program: _____

_____

narrative: _____

_____

nontherapeutic research: _____

_____

obliterate: _____

_____

patient information: _____

_____

personal information: _____

_____

problem-oriented medical record (POMR) charting: _____

_____

progress notes: _____

_____

purge: _____

_____

SOAP note charting: _____

_____

social information: _____

_____

source-oriented medical record: _____

_____

standard of care: _____

_____

statute of limitations: _____

_____

subpoena: _____

_____

ABBREVIATIONS

Provide the meanings of the following abbreviations:

EDP: _____

EHR: _____

FDA: _____

© 2015 Pearson Education, Inc.

HIPAA: _____

NKA: _____

PHI: _____

POMR: _____

SOAP: _____

SOMR: _____

CRITICAL THINKING QUESTIONS

1. Lily Foote, CMA (AAMA), is working with Dr. Marla Tiffany. Dr. Tiffany has asked Lily to create a policy for how medical records will be handled for patients who are involved in the medical research programs in which Dr. Tiffany participates. How should Lily proceed?

_____

_____

_____

_____

_____

2. Susan Haufe, CMAS (AMT), is working with a small, one-doctor internal medicine clinic. The physician, Dr. Chentow, is retiring and will not be transferring his files to another physician. How should Susan proceed with working with the patient files that are in the office?

_____

_____

_____

_____

3. Rodney Jarvis is in an administrative medical assisting class. He has been given an assignment to create a policy for documenting prescription refill requests in the medical office. What might Rodney create?

_____

_____

_____

_____

4. Michael Manson, RMA (AMT), has just been hired to work in a family practice clinic. On his first day in the office, he notices that many patient charts have words such as *problem* and *talker* listed on them. He asks the MA who is training him about these words and is told it is the office's way of noting those patients who are difficult to work with or who talk excessively during their visit. What kinds of problems might this facility encounter when using these notations?

_____

_____

_____

_____

_____

_____

5. Chris Nichols, CMA (AAMA), has been given the task of deciding which patient files to purge from the clinic in order to create more storage room. How should Chris proceed with this project?

_____

_____

_____

_____

_____

CHAPTER REVIEW TEST

MULTIPLE CHOICE

Circle the letter of the correct answer.

1. Which of the following techniques is the appropriate way to correct an error in the patient's medical record?
   a. Use white correction fluid to obliterate the error.
   b. Use a black marker to obliterate the error.
   c. Draw a single line through the error, initial and date the correction.
   d. Scribble it out.
   e. None of the above

2. Under which of the following circumstances can the patient's medical record be copied and released?
   a. When the patient's spouse comes to the office to request a copy
   b. When the patient's employer calls the office to request a copy
   c. When the office receives a subpoena signed by a judge requesting a copy
   d. When the patient's brother sends in a letter asking for a copy
   e. All of the above

3. Medicare guidelines dictate that patient medical records must be kept in the office for at least _____ years from the patient's last date of service.
   a. 5
   b. 10
   c. 15
   d. 20
   e. 25

© 2015 Pearson Education, Inc.

4. Once an office is out of room for storing patient medical records, which of the following is an appropriate way to store them?
   a. Scan the record and record it onto a CD.
   b. Scan the record and record it onto a DVD.
   c. Scan the record and record it on microfilm.
   d. Scan the record and record it on microfiche.
   e. All of the above

5. Which of the following is true about retaining patient medical records?
   a. The record should be kept for 3 years from the date of the last service.
   b. The length of time the record is kept is determined by the statute of limitations in any particular state.
   c. The record should be kept until the patient reaches age 18.
   d. The record should be kept for 5 years from the date of the last service.
   e. The record should be kept for 7 years from the date of the last service.

6. _____ patient files are the files of patients who have moved and will not be continuing to treat with the physician or facility.
   a. Open
   b. Closed
   c. Inactive
   d. Purged
   e. Discontinued

7. _____ patient files are the files of patients who have not been in to see the physician for a period of between 2 and 5 years, depending upon the type of practice.
   a. Open
   b. Closed
   c. Inactive
   d. Purged
   e. Discontinued

8. _____ patient files are the files of patients who have been in to see the physician recently.
   a. Open
   b. Closed
   c. Inactive
   d. Purged
   e. Discontinued

9. Which of the following is a situation where the medical office might use a flow chart to track patient care?
   a. To track an infant's weight and length
   b. To chart appropriate patient telephone calls
   c. To chart needed patient medical procedures
   d. To chart a patient's record of payments
   e. To chart the number of times a patient visits the medical practice in the course of a year

10. _____ are a type of medical charting that tracks a patient's problems throughout medical care by assigning a number to each of the patient's medical problems.
    a. Narrative notes
    b. SOAP notes
    c. POMR notes
    d. CHEDDAR notes
    e. SOMR notes

TRUE/FALSE

Identify whether the statement is true (T) or false (F).

_____ 1. The FDA requires extensive testing before drugs are considered safe and effective enough to be released.

_____ 2. If the physician does NOT authorize a prescription refill request, it does not need to be documented in the patient's medical record.

_____ 3. Medical offices should have a policy that requires a minimum of 24 hours for prescription refill requests.

_____ 4. The medical record belongs to the physician or facility, whereas the information contained within the medical record belongs to the patient.

_____ 5. Paper medical records can be converted to an electronic format for long-term storage.

_____ 6. After converting paper medical records to an electronic format, the medical office should shred the original record.

_____ 7. Filing patients numerically can be considered more secure than filing patients alphabetically.

_____ 8. Using abbreviations in the medical chart can lead to confusion or errors in patient care.

_____ 9. Anytime a medical record contains a signature with initials rather than the signer's full name, the medical office must keep a permanent record of the signer.

_____ 10. Some health care providers may review patient medical records as part of consultation visits or "second opinions."

SHORT ANSWER

1. What is meant by *nontherapeutic research*?

   _____
   _____
   _____
   _____
   _____

2. Describe how to accurately make a late entry addition to the patient's medical record.

   _____
   _____
   _____
   _____
   _____

3. Explain why the medical assistant needs to know the state statute of limitations for malpractice lawsuits when considering how long to keep a patient's medical record.

   _____
   _____
   _____
   _____
   _____

© 2015 Pearson Education, Inc.

4. Describe the steps a medical assistant might take to locate a misfiled patient file in the medical office.

_____

_____

_____

_____

5. Explain why a medical office may opt for filing patients numerically as opposed to alphabetically.

_____

_____

_____

_____

6. Describe the CHEDDAR form of charting.

_____

_____

_____

_____

7. Describe SOAP note charting. Why is this method of charting popular in medical offices?

_____

_____

_____

_____

8. Give three examples of patient telephone calls that would need to be charted in the patient's medical record.

_____

_____

_____

_____

9. Give three examples of patient telephone calls that would *not* need to be charted in the patient's medical record.

_____

_____

_____

_____

10. Describe the five Cs of charting.

_____

_____

_____

_____

CHAPTER 12
Electronic Health Records

CHAPTER OUTLINE

COMPETENCY SKILLS PERFORMANCE

CHAPTER REVIEW

- The term *electronic health record* refers to a patient's entire medical history in electronic form. Electronic health records are kept on a computer's hard drive or a medical office's computer network rather than on paper.

- The term *electronic medical record* (EMR) refers to the medical information collected on the patient in one particular physician's office.

- Electronic health records offer enhanced ease, efficiency, and accessibility. Keeping records in paper form may cause storage difficulties as well as issues in keeping patient information confidential.

- In 2009, Congress passed the Health Information Technology for Economic and Clinical Health Act, also known as the HITECH Act. This legislation provided access to incentive payments to physicians, with the goal of increasing the use of electronic health record systems in physician practices. In order to qualify for the incentives for providing an electronic health record under this legislation, the electronic health record used by physicians had to meet specific meaningful use objectives.

- With paper charting, the patient's chart is only available to one staff member at a time. Electronic health records make the patient's chart available to many health care team members at the same time.

- The conversion from paper to electronic health record format is typically done over time. Once paper medical records are converted to electronic versions, those paper records must be appropriately destroyed.

- Medical offices should correct errors in a patient chart according to accepted protocol.

© 2015 Pearson Education, Inc.

- By using electronic health records, a medical office is able to perform tasks such as sending reminder postcards more easily than performing these same tasks with paper medical records.
- Other benefits of electronic health records include using electronic signatures, avoiding medical mistakes, saving time, and communicating between staff members.
- Meaningful use is an incentive program put into place by the CMS to promote the use of electronic health records in medical facilities.

LEARNING ACTIVITIES

To ensure that you have achieved the learning objectives in this chapter:

1. In the Terminology Review section on page 108, define the key terminology found in this chapter of your student text.

2. Create a list of steps to take to complete an electronic health record.

_____
_____
_____
_____
_____
_____
_____
_____
_____

3. Create a list of steps to take to correct a mistake in the electronic health record.

_____
_____
_____
_____
_____
_____
_____
_____
_____
_____

APPLIED LEARNING EXERCISES

Using a separate sheet of paper, complete the following assignments:

1. Using the Internet as a research source, locate three companies that sell electronic health records software. Create a list of the pros and cons of each system.

2. Write a brief essay that identifies the steps to take to properly destroy a paper medical record after it has been converted to an electronic health record.

TERMINOLOGY REVIEW

Using the glossary and highlighted terms in the textbook, define the following terms:

electronic health record: _____

_____

electronic signature: _____

_____

indecipherable: _____

_____

meaningful use: _____

_____

_____

ABBREVIATIONS

Provide the meanings of the following abbreviations:

CMS: _____

EHR: _____

EMR: _____

HIPAA: _____

HITECH Act: _____

CRITICAL THINKING QUESTIONS

1. Rosa Valdez, CMA (AAMA), is working in the billing office in a urology practice. The office uses electronic health records for patient charting. Rosa frequently finds that she needs to alert other staff members about her need to speak with a patient about his or her account. How might Rosa devise a way to alert her coworkers of the need to see a patient when the patient comes into the office?

   _____

   _____

   _____

   _____

   _____

2. Chris Hernandez, RMA (AMT), is the office manager of a busy family practice clinic. Chris has been asked by the physicians to come up with some ideas for using the electronic health records software to create a marketing program. What kinds of ideas could Chris suggest for this project?

   _____

   _____

   _____

   _____

   _____

   _____

© 2015 Pearson Education, Inc.

3. Mickey Cape is taking a course on electronic health records. Mickey has been given an assignment to write a policy on how to dispose of paper medical records once a record has been converted to electronic form. What might Mickey come up with?

_____

_____

_____

_____

_____

4. Barret Risenhour, CMAS (AMT), is the office manager in a women's clinic. The physicians in the clinic are considering moving to electronic health records from the paper records they have been using for years. Barret has been asked to create a list of the functions of an electronic health record system. What might Barret's list contain?

_____

_____

_____

_____

_____

5. Dr. Shawn Hagen has been using paper medical records in his practice for over 20 years. He is reluctant to change to electronic health records because he feels his computer skills are poor. What sort of information can his office manager give to him about the ease of converting from paper to electronic health records?

_____

_____

_____

_____

_____

CHAPTER REVIEW TEST

MULTIPLE CHOICE

Circle the letter of the correct answer.

1. Some clinics allow patients to access the clinic's network or intranet. What are these patients able to do with this type of password-protected system access?
   a. Review their lab results
   b. Review their record of immunizations
   c. Review their medication levels
   d. Schedule an appointment
   e. All of the above

2. Which of the following diagnostic tests can be performed with electronic health records and testing equipment?
   a. Digital X-rays
   b. Holter monitors
   c. Spirometers
   d. Lab tests on blood and urine samples
   e. All of the above

3. Which of the following tasks do many health care providers believe they spend more time doing?
   a. Charting in the patient's medical record
   b. Working with the patient in person
   c. Writing prescriptions for patients
   d. Cleaning the medical office
   e. Ordering administrative supplies

4. Which state passed a law in March 2006 requiring health care providers to submit prescriptions electronically or print them, rather than using cursive writing?
   a. Idaho
   b. Montana
   c. New York
   d. Washington
   e. California

5. At least _____ people, and perhaps many more, die in hospitals every year as a result of medical mistakes that could have been prevented.
   a. 25,000
   b. 38,000
   c. 44,000
   d. 52,000
   e. 90,000

6. Which of the following functions are commonly found within an electronic health record?
   a. Time stamp recordings
   b. The ability to fax prescriptions to the pharmacy
   c. The ability to attach digital photos to the patient's record
   d. Electronically ordered lab results, imaging items, or medical tests
   e. All of the above

7. Many medical offices use PDAs to record information into the patient's medical record. What does the acronym PDA stand for?
   a. Private data access
   b. Personal digital assistant
   c. Personal data assistant
   d. Private data assets
   e. Personal data access

8. How often should a backup of the medical office computer system be done?
   a. Every hour
   b. Twice per day
   c. Once a day
   d. Once a week
   e. Once a month

9. In keeping in compliance with _____ legislation, all computer users in the medical office must have their own password and login.
   a. TJC
   b. CLIA
   c. OSHA
   d. HIPAA
   e. HITECH

10. Which of the following members of the medical office team should attend training sessions for using electronic health record software?
   a. The office manager
   b. The receptionist
   c. The physician
   d. The administrative medical assistant
   e. All of the above

© 2015 Pearson Education, Inc.

TRUE/FALSE

Identify whether the statement is true (T) or false (F).

_____ 1. Electronic health records offer enhanced ease, efficiency, and accessibility.

_____ 2. Using electronic health records, a medical office can send reminder postcards to patients more easily than performing this task using paper medical records.

_____ 3. The Health Information Technology for Economic and Clinical Health Act of 2009, also known as the HITECH Act, is legislation that provided access to incentive payments to physicians, with the goal of increasing the use of electronic health record systems in physician practices.

_____ 4. Computer users can share passwords used to access patient medical records.

_____ 5. Once the medical office has converted from paper to electronic health records, the paper medical record should be stored in the medical office.

_____ 6. Most electronic health records programs have drop-down menus that allow the user to choose information from a list.

_____ 7. It is believed that some medical errors are caused by indecipherable handwriting.

_____ 8. Using electronic health records, health care providers may be alerted to possible medication errors.

_____ 9. In medical offices where electronic signatures are used, an original version of the user's signature must be kept on file in the office.

_____ 10. All medical facilities use the same software for electronic health records.

SHORT ANSWER

1. Explain the steps to take to make a correction in the electronic health record.

   _____
   _____
   _____
   _____

2. Outline the benefits to patients when the medical office allows them to access portions of their electronic health records via the Internet.

   _____
   _____
   _____
   _____

3. Create a list of health maintenance reminders a medical office might send to its patients.

   _____
   _____
   _____

4. Explain how using electronic health records eases the process of sending patient medical information to the patient's health insurance company.

_____

_____

_____

_____

5. What are the benefits of having all staff members, including the physicians, train on the use of electronic health records?

_____

_____

_____

_____

6. Describe the HITECH Act of 2009.

_____

_____

_____

_____

7. Define *meaningful use* as it pertains to the use of electronic health records.

_____

_____

_____

_____

8. List two safeguards medical offices should employ to ensure patient confidentiality when using electronic health records.

_____

_____

_____

_____

9. What are the benefits of allowing more than one person in the medical office to access the patient's electronic health record at the same time?

_____

_____

_____

_____

© 2015 Pearson Education, Inc.

10. Describe the process to follow to back up computers and electronic health records. Why is it important to follow this process?

_____

_____

_____

_____

_____

© 2015 Pearson Education, Inc.

CHAPTER 13
Computers in the Medical Office

CHAPTER OUTLINE

COMPETENCY SKILLS PERFORMANCE

CHAPTER REVIEW

- Computers are used in the medical office to perform a variety of functions, ranging from billing and coding to appointment scheduling to managing inventory of supplies.

- Computers consist of hardware (the equipment itself), software that is used to perform the needed functions in the medical office, and the peripherals that attach to the computer system to perform tasks such as backing up data or printing documents.

- In order to remain compliant with HIPAA legislation with regard to patient privacy, all computers in the medical office must be password-protected and must have safeguards in place to keep unauthorized persons from gaining access to private patient information.

- Office staff can take steps to maintain computer equipment, but repairs should be left to professionals.

- Medical offices will have a printer attached to the computer to allow the printing of documents from within the software. Many offices will also have a scanner attached to the computer to allow health care professionals to scan a document and add it into the computer's software program.

© 2015 Pearson Education, Inc.

- The Internet can serve as a resource for nearly infinite amounts of medical information.
- Medical offices should state clear policies for the use of their computers.
- Many physicians today use personal digital assistants and smart phones to quickly check dosages or research drug interactions.
- Ergonomically designed computer equipment helps ensure that all members of the health care team work safely.

LEARNING ACTIVITIES

To ensure that you have achieved the learning objectives in this chapter:

1. In the Terminology Review section on page 116, define the key terminology found in this chapter of your student text.

2. Imagine you have been asked to research the price of purchasing a new computer for the medical office. Create a list of the steps you would take to determine the type of system best for the office.

3. Create a list of suggestions for securing office computers from unauthorized access.

4. Describe a personal digital assistant, including how this device can be used with electronic medical software.

APPLIED LEARNING EXERCISES

Using a separate sheet of paper, complete the following assignments:

1. Using the Internet as a research source, locate two companies that sell electronic pads and tablets. Create a list of pros and cons associated with purchasing this equipment from each of these vendors.

2. Create an office policy for how to properly maintain computer equipment.

3. Create an office policy for staff personal use of the computers in the medical office.

4. Write a brief essay that explains the basic principles of computer ergonomics. Describe how the administrative medical assistant can use computer ergonomics to avoid injury in the medical office.

TERMINOLOGY REVIEW

Using the glossary and highlighted terms in the textbook, define the following terms:

bar-code scanner: _____

_____

battery backup system: _____

_____

computer peripherals: _____

_____

computer virus: _____

_____

electronic sign-in sheet: _____

_____

ergonomic: _____

_____

flash drive: _____

_____

health-related calculator: _____

_____

Internet search engine: _____

_____

malware: _____

_____

medical management software: _____

_____

personal digital assistant: _____

_____

scanner: _____

_____

smart phone: _____

_____

thumb drive: _____

_____

ABBREVIATIONS

Provide the meanings of the following abbreviations:

AMA: _____

CD: _____

CDC: _____

© 2015 Pearson Education, Inc.

CPU: _____

DPI: _____

DVD: _____

FDA: _____

HIPAA: _____

PDA: _____

PHI: _____

RAM: _____

ROM: _____

URL: _____

USB: _____

VIPPS: _____

CRITICAL THINKING QUESTIONS

1. Marcia Dukat, CMA (AAMA), is the administrative medical assistant at the River Valley Health Clinic. The physician, Dr. Andrew Smith, would like the clinical staff to use portable electronic pads and tablets while in the patient care area so that they can enter information into patient charts without the need to be connected physically to the computer. He assigns Marcia the task of researching and working with an electronic tablet company to set this up in the office. How would Marcia explain to the office staff how the electronic pads and tablets will work in the daily operations of the office?

_____

_____

_____

_____

_____

_____

2. Tanya Brown, RMA (AMT), is discussing the need for a new computer system with the physician. Dr. Benton has asked Tanya to describe the difference among the hardware, the software, and the peripherals that go with various computer systems. How might Tanya define these three components?

_____

_____

_____

_____

3. Wanda Vallone, NCMA (NCCT), is an administrative medical assistant at the Pineview Women's Health Clinic. Because Wanda often forgets her computer password, she has written it down on a sticky note and taped it to her computer. In addition, Wanda often fails to log out of her computer when her workstation is unattended. How should the office manager address these potential computer security issues?

_____

_____

_____

© 2015 Pearson Education, Inc.   *Computers in the Medical Office*   **117**

_____

_____

_____

4. George El Fashir, CMA (AAMA), has been asked to describe the various computer drives that might be used to store information from the computer systems in his office. What information should George prepare?

_____

_____

_____

_____

_____

5. Gene Armand, CMAA (NHA), is training a new administrative medical assistant on the use of the office's computer system. He warns the new MA to be wary of opening e-mail attachments from unknown senders and of downloading certain files from the Internet. What might be the danger in doing these things, and how might the office protect itself from potential damage?

_____

_____

_____

_____

_____

_____

CHAPTER REVIEW TEST

MULTIPLE CHOICE

Circle the letter of the correct answer.

1. _____ are devices that allow documents to be copied and transferred into the computer system.
   a. Thumb drives
   b. Personal digital assistants
   c. Printers
   d. Scanners
   e. Smart phones

2. The higher a monitor's DPI, _____.
   a. the clearer its picture
   b. the faster its Internet access
   c. the less it costs
   d. the more computer peripherals that can be attached to it
   e. None of the above

3. The _____ is the computer equipment.
   a. hardware
   b. software
   c. peripheral
   d. USB
   e. thumb drive

© 2015 Pearson Education, Inc.

4. Malware includes all of the following EXCEPT _____.
   a. Norton
   b. worms
   c. spyware
   d. adware
   e. Trojan horses

5. _____ are used for large-volume applications such as government statistics.
   a. Supercomputers
   b. Mainframe computers
   c. Minicomputers
   d. Microcomputers
   e. Personal digital assistants

6. Which of the following is a popular search engine used to retrieve information from the Internet?
   a. Yahoo!
   b. Google
   c. Bing
   d. Dog Pile
   e. All of the above

7. The computer's CPU is considered the computer's _____.
   a. memory
   b. brain
   c. keyboard
   d. mouse
   e. peripheral

8. An ergonomic keyboard is used to _____.
   a. reduce typing stress by supporting the hands and wrists comfortably
   b. connect to the computer via a wireless connection
   c. type faster than using a conventional keyboard
   d. maintain patient privacy when using the keyboard
   e. None of the above

9. Which of the following is a small, mobile handheld device that provides computing and information storage retrieval capabilities for personal or business use?
   a. Personal digital assistant
   b. Minicomputer
   c. Microcomputer
   d. Laptop
   e. Mainframe computer

10. Many physicians today use _____ to quickly check medication dosages and to research drug interactions.
    a. mainframes
    b. supercomputers
    c. main computers
    d. smart phones
    e. minicomputers

TRUE/FALSE

Identify whether the statement is true (T) or false (F).

_____ 1. DVDs are made of a thin metal.

_____ 2. A flash drive is sometimes called a thumb drive.

_____ 3. Flash drives typically connect to the computer via a USB port.

_____ 4. With regard to external storage devices, the larger the amount of storage available, the higher the cost.

_____ 5. RAM is used to store media that are not easily modified.

_____ 6. When a computer's RAM is insufficient, the computer typically runs slower.

_____ 7. When determining the type of printer an office should purchase, one consideration is the cost of the supplies.

_____ 8. All medical offices should have a battery backup system to protect data from loss.

_____ 9. HIPAA legislation requires medical office computers to be password-protected.

_____ 10. An electronic sign-in sheet is an example of a computer peripheral.

SHORT ANSWER

1. Describe how a scanner might be used in the medical office.

_____

_____

_____

_____

2. Describe how a digital camera might be used in the medical office.

_____

_____

_____

_____

3. Why might a medical office use a bar code scanner?

_____

_____

_____

_____

4. Describe how a medical office might use a sign-in sheet while still remaining HIPAA compliant.

_____

_____

_____

_____

5. Why is it important for the medical office to institute a policy regarding personal use of office computers?

_____

_____

_____

© 2015 Pearson Education, Inc.

6. List the various features commonly found in medical management software.

_____

_____

_____

_____

_____

7. What type of support should come with the purchase of medical office management software?

_____

_____

_____

_____

_____

8. List the HIPAA safeguards for safeguarding protected health information.

_____

_____

_____

_____

_____

9. List six Internet search engines that may be used to search for data.

_____

_____

_____

_____

_____

10. List six medical organizations whose Web sites could be used to find the latest information on research, medications, and techniques.

_____

_____

_____

_____

CHAPTER 14
Equipment, Maintenance, and Supply Inventory

CHAPTER OUTLINE

COMPETENCY SKILLS PERFORMANCE

CHAPTER REVIEW

- Every medical office must have a system in place for maintaining equipment and for keeping track of supplies in an efficient manner.

- Medical office equipment is quite often very expensive and must be maintained according to manufacturers' directions.

- An equipment maintenance manual serves to ensure all needed equipment is in working order and able to support business initiatives.

- Any employee who uses equipment in the medical office must be trained to use the equipment in a way that provides both for the safety of the employee and for the proper use of the equipment.

- There are distinct advantages both to leasing and to buying office equipment. Physicians may choose one option over the other based upon the clinic's needs at the time of acquiring the equipment.

© 2015 Pearson Education, Inc.

- Faxing documents in the medical office requires strict attention to patient confidentiality. Whenever confidential documents must be faxed, a HIPAA-compliant fax cover sheet must be used.
- Staff in the medical office often become adept at using 10-key calculators to manipulate numbers.
- Most medical transcription is done outside of the medical office. Frequently, transcription is done by persons working outside of the United States. When using an offshore service, the medical facility must be certain the transcription company abides by HIPAA legislation and properly protects patient confidentiality.
- An inventory control manual helps a medical office ensure that it is always fully equipped with needed supplies.
- Medical office supplies are typically split into two categories—administrative and clinical. Clinical supplies will generally be ordered from suppliers and may take several days to acquire. Administrative supplies may be ordered from local office supply stores.
- Every medical office should have a system in place for inventorying all office supplies. This system should include policies for how to order supplies, how to stock supplies when they arrive in the office, and how to discard supplies that have gone beyond their expiration date. Drug samples must be tracked, and notice must be taken of any expiration dates on these samples.

LEARNING ACTIVITIES

To ensure that you have achieved the learning objectives in this chapter:

1. In the Terminology Review section on page 124, define the key terminology found in this chapter of your student text.
2. List the pros and cons of leasing or purchasing equipment for the medical office.

_____

_____

_____

_____

_____

3. Write a brief essay describing the purpose and importance of an equipment training manual.

_____

_____

_____

_____

_____

APPLIED LEARNING EXERCISES

Using a separate sheet of paper, complete the following assignments:

1. Create an office equipment maintenance manual.
2. Using the Internet as a research source, search for three computer equipment vendors. Create a list of the pros and cons of purchasing from each of these companies.
3. Create an office policy for maintaining patient confidentiality while using the fax machine in the medical office.

4. Write a brief essay describing the use of outside transcription services. Be sure to include the pros and cons for using services that are located outside of the United States.

5. Create an inventory control manual that could be used in the medical office.

TERMINOLOGY REVIEW

Using the glossary and highlighted terms in the textbook, define the following terms:

expiration date: _____

_____

inventory: _____

_____

maintained: _____

_____

packing slip: _____

_____

scanner: _____

_____

transcribe: _____

_____

transcription machine: _____

_____

user manual: _____

_____

warranty: _____

_____

ABBREVIATIONS

Provide the meanings of the following abbreviations:

HIPAA: _____

OSHA: _____

CRITICAL THINKING QUESTIONS

1. Corey Steinberg, CMA (AAMA), has recently been hired to work as an administrative medical assistant in a busy cardiology practice. Corey has been given the task of creating a manual that outlines the warranty information as well as the maintenance schedule for each piece of medical office equipment. How should Corey go about beginning this task?

_____

_____

_____

© 2015 Pearson Education, Inc.

_____

_____

_____

2. Monte Beaton, RMA (AMT), is the office manager in a gastroenterology practice. Monte has recently hired three new medical assistants and wants to be sure they are properly trained to use each piece of equipment in the medical office. How can Monte be sure the training is done properly?

_____

_____

_____

_____

_____

_____

3. Krystle Shawger is taking an administrative class as part of her medical assisting training. She has been given an assignment to write a brief essay describing how an equipment maintenance log would be useful in the medical office. What might Krystle include in her paper?

_____

_____

_____

_____

_____

_____

4. Marian Harrison, RMA (AMT), is the administrative office manager in a family practice clinic. She is writing an office policy for inventorying administrative office equipment. What might her policy include?

_____

_____

_____

_____

_____

5. Joann Felmer, CMA (AAMA), works in a walk-in clinic. At the weekly office staff meeting, the office manager mentioned the need for purchasing a new ECG machine. The office manager has asked Joann to research the various options available. How should Joann handle this task?

_____

_____

_____

_____

_____

CHAPTER REVIEW TEST

MULTIPLE CHOICE

Circle the letter of the correct answer.

1. When researching new office equipment, which of the following is an appropriate avenue for the medical assistant in determining the best equipment for the office to purchase?
   a. Ask the vendor to bring the equipment to the office for a demonstration.
   b. Call other medical offices that are using the equipment.
   c. Go to stores where the equipment is being sold to look at the equipment.
   d. Research the equipment on the Internet.
   e. All of the above

2. Which of the following is an advantage of leasing over buying a piece of equipment?
   a. Little or no money is required at the time of acquiring the equipment.
   b. The medical office owns the equipment.
   c. The equipment repair is not covered by the manufacturer.
   d. A down payment is required.
   e. The employer is responsible for all training.

3. Which of the following is an appropriate place for the fax machine to be located in the medical office?
   a. In the reception room
   b. In a treatment room
   c. In the billing office
   d. In the hallway
   e. None of the above

4. When the medical office needs to send confidential patient information to another medical facility, which of the following is the most secure way to do so?
   a. Send the documents via fax.
   b. Send the document via courier.
   c. Send the document via the postal service.
   d. Send the document attached to an e-mail.
   e. Send the document via FedEx.

5. When faxing a document from the medical office, which of the following pieces of information should be included on the fax cover sheet?
   a. The name of the clinic sending the document
   b. The name of the clinic receiving the document
   c. The number of pages included in the fax
   d. Personal name
   e. All of the above

6. Which of the following considerations should be made when researching possible copy machines to purchase for the medical office?
   a. The cost of supplies for the copier
   b. The price of the copier
   c. The warranty associated with the copier
   d. The availability and cost of replacement parts
   e. All of the above

© 2015 Pearson Education, Inc.

7. When researching outside transcription services, what is the most important consideration the medical office must make?

 a. The cost of the transcription service
 b. The speed with which the service will return transcribed documents
 c. Whether the transcription company is HIPAA-compliant
 d. The availability of the transcription company to come to the medical office in person
 e. All of the above

8. In order to effectively keep track of medical office supplies, which of the following should be included in the list of inventory?

 a. The name of the supply
 b. The order or part number
 c. The name of the company who supplies the item
 d. The typical quantity and frequency of ordering
 e. All of the above

9. In order to effectively manage office inventory, how often should the medical office perform inventory?

 a. Daily
 b. Weekly
 c. Monthly
 d. Yearly
 e. This will vary; it depends upon the needs of the office.

10. What information should be included on the packing slip that comes with a shipment of supplies?

 a. A list of the supplies included in the shipment
 b. A list of supplies that may be ordered in the future
 c. A list of upcoming sales or promotions the supplier is advertising
 d. All of the above
 e. None of the above

TRUE/FALSE

Identify whether the statement is true (T) or false (F).

_____ 1. The packing slip that comes with supply shipments may also serve as an invoice.

_____ 2. If part of an order is missing or back-ordered when a supply shipment is received, the medical assistant should file the packing slip with the paid invoices.

_____ 3. All office supplies should be stored with the newest supplies to be used first.

_____ 4. It is illegal to use expired medical supplies.

_____ 5. Pharmaceutical companies often supply physicians with drug samples in the hope those physicians will prescribe the drugs.

_____ 6. Drug samples have expiration dates.

_____ 7. Medical offices should track drug samples in order to discourage staff from taking drugs for personal use.

_____ 8. According to the USDA, the proper way to dispose of medications is to remove the medicine from its container, mix it with an undesirable substance in a plastic bag, and then discard in the trash.

_____ 9. Clerical supplies are easier to stock than clinical supplies.

_____ 10. Many medical offices use computer software to track supplies.

SHORT ANSWER

1. Explain how an equipment maintenance manual benefits the medical office.

   _____

   _____

   _____

   _____

   _____

2. Describe a 10-key calculator and its function in the medical office.

   _____

   _____

   _____

   _____

   _____

3. Describe how transcription machines worked in years past.

   _____

   _____

   _____

   _____

   _____

4. How should the medical office maintain patient confidentiality when using the fax machine?

   _____

   _____

   _____

   _____

   _____

5. Why are clerical supplies easier to stock than medical supplies?

   _____

   _____

   _____

   _____

6. How should expired drugs be handled in the medical office?

   _____

   _____

   _____

   _____

   _____

© 2015 Pearson Education, Inc.

7. Describe the steps to take when receiving a supply shipment.

_____

_____

_____

_____

_____

8. Explain why medical office staff would check for needed supplies for the next day before leaving the office the night before.

_____

_____

_____

_____

_____

9. When a medical office discovers a supplier offering low prices for quantity purchases, what should the medical assistant consider before purchasing a large quantity of any given supply?

_____

_____

_____

_____

_____

10. Where in the medical office should the office copier and fax machine *not* be located?

_____

_____

_____

_____

_____

CHAPTER 15

Office Policies and Procedures

CHAPTER OUTLINE

COMPETENCY SKILLS PERFORMANCE

Procedure 15-1: Create an Office Brochure

Procedure 15-2: Create a Procedure for the Procedure Manual

CHAPTER REVIEW

- Many medical offices use informational pamphlets to convey information to and educate patients. Whereas some clinics purchase these pamphlets in a ready-made form from suppliers, other offices design and create their own pamphlets.

- Office personnel manuals ensure that all members of the health care team perform appropriately and to consistent standards. Personnel policies are those surrounding employment information, such as health insurance benefits or vacation time off. These policies should be clearly written and must be fairly applied to all employees in the office.

- A policies and procedures manual in the medical office serves as a written record of the legal, desired behavior of all health care staff. When employees clearly understand the office policies and are given a written example of how procedures in the office are to be handled, training of new employees takes less time, and there is less confusion among staff members.

- In larger offices, administrative policies may be housed in a separate manual from those policies addressing clinical areas. Per Occupational Safety and Health Administration (OSHA) regulations, infection control and quality improvement and risk management procedures must be kept in separate notebooks and reviewed and updated regularly.

LEARNING ACTIVITY

In the Terminology Review section on page 131, define the key terminology found in this chapter of your student text.

© 2015 Pearson Education, Inc.

APPLIED LEARNING EXERCISES

Using a separate sheet of paper, complete the following assignments:

1. Create a patient information pamphlet.
2. Using the Internet as a research source, research the type of personnel policies that might be found in a medical office. Create a list of 10 policies you find, and explain how each would be useful in the medical office.
3. Create 10 policies or procedures that might be used in a manual for a medical office.

TERMINOLOGY REVIEW

Using the glossary and highlighted terms in the textbook, define the following terms:

brochure: _____

_____

mission statement: _____

_____

organizational chart: _____

_____

personnel manual: _____

_____

policy: _____

_____

procedure: _____

_____

ABBREVIATIONS

Provide the meanings of the following abbreviations:

HIPAA: _____

OSHA: _____

CRITICAL THINKING QUESTIONS

1. Macy Goldsmith is taking an administrative medical assisting class. She has been asked to design and create an informational pamphlet that could be given to a patient in a health care setting. What should Macy consider before starting this project? What should she include?

_____

_____

_____

_____

_____

_____

2. Hiro Yoshi, CMA (AAMA), has recently been hired to work in a busy walk-in clinic. Hiro wants to find out what the office policy is regarding taking time off after the birth of a new child. He doesn't want to ask his coworkers or the office manager because he doesn't want his new employer to know he and his wife are trying to have a baby. How can Hiro find this information without having to discuss the issue with his coworkers?

---

3. Larry Anderson, CMAS (AMT), has been working for Dr. Bacon for 7 years. Last year he asked to take time off over the July Fourth holiday. At that time, Larry was told the office did not allow time off over holidays. The office personnel policy manual confirms this is the office policy. Sara Hastings, RMA (AMT), has just been hired by Dr. Bacon. Larry overhears Sara ask for time off over the upcoming Memorial Day weekend. The office manager grants Sara her request. What can Larry do about this seemingly unfair application of the office policy regarding time off over holidays?

---

4. Julie Ryan, CMA (AAMA), is the office manager in a busy urology practice. The clinic has an office policy manual, but it has not been updated in over 10 years. As Julie looks through the manual, she sees several policies that are outdated and no longer apply to the office. How should Julie go about the process of updating her clinic policy manual?

---

5. Beth Watanabe, RMA (AMT), is the office manager in a pediatric clinic. Joe Jensen, NCMA (NCCT), was hired to work in this clinic 1 month ago. Though Joe wore appropriate attire, including clean scrubs and shoes at the beginning of his employment, he has been gradually moving away from the office dress code policy and has recently been wearing street clothes and open-toed shoes to work. Beth has asked Joe to wear the appropriate attire, but Joe says he doesn't see why he should have to dress so blandly. What can Beth do to address this situation?

© 2015 Pearson Education, Inc.

CHAPTER REVIEW TEST

MULTIPLE CHOICE

Circle the letter of the correct answer.

1. Which of the following is an example of an administrative office policy?
   a. The steps to handling a missed patient appointment
   b. The steps to cleaning the exam room tables
   c. The steps to processing lab specimens
   d. The steps to administering ear medication
   e. The steps to administering CPR

2. Which of the following is an example of a clinical office policy?
   a. The steps to handling a missed patient appointment
   b. The steps to cleaning the exam room tables
   c. The steps to processing lab specimens
   d. The steps to processing an insurance claim
   e. The steps to researching a diagnosis code

3. Which of the following is an example of a risk management office policy?
   a. The steps to handling a missed patient appointment
   b. The steps to cleaning the exam room tables
   c. The steps to processing lab specimens
   d. The steps to escorting patients while in the medical office
   e. The steps to reducing patient wait time while on the telephone

4. Which of the following is an example of a personnel policy?
   a. Jury duty
   b. Medical insurance benefits
   c. Dental insurance benefits
   d. Sick leave policy
   e. All of the above

5. Which of the following is an example of a quality improvement policy?
   a. Decreasing patient wait times for appointments
   b. Jury duty
   c. Family medical leave time
   d. Personal use of the telephone in the medical office
   e. Personal use of medical office computers

6. How often should the office policy and procedures manual be updated?
   a. Weekly
   b. Monthly
   c. Bimonthly
   d. Yearly
   e. As needed

7. According to _____, quality improvement and risk management procedures must be kept in a separate notebook that is clearly marked and updated regularly.
   a. TJC
   b. HIPAA
   c. OSHA
   d. CDC
   e. FDA

8. According to _____, the infection control procedures manual must be kept separate from other procedure manuals in the office.

   a. TJC
   b. HIPAA
   c. OSHA

   d. CDC
   e. FDA

9. Which of the following is an example of an infection control procedure?

   a. Employee needlestick injuries
   b. Decreasing patient wait times for appointments

   c. Jury duty
   d. Family medical leave time
   e. Sick leave policy

10. A policy regarding releasing medical information to a patient is an example of what kind of policy?

   a. Clinical
   b. Infection control
   c. Risk management

   d. Administrative
   e. Quality improvement

TRUE/FALSE

Identify whether the statement is true (T) or false (F).

_____ 1. Any clinical procedure that requires intervention should be documented for employee reference.

_____ 2. One of the most important reasons for having a medical office policy and procedures manual is to clarify rules and regulations and the physician's expectations for procedures.

_____ 3. A grievance procedure policy addresses how employees should handle situations in which they disagree with their supervisor.

_____ 4. For all material in an office policy and procedures manual, it is important to keep only state laws in mind to ensure all policies are within legal boundaries.

_____ 5. Office brochures are a useful way to educate patients on the physician's specific types of treatment or therapy.

_____ 6. Every member of the health care team is responsible for educating patients.

_____ 7. Policies and procedures are not as important in the medical field as in other fields.

_____ 8. A procedure is a statement of guidelines or rules on a given topic.

_____ 9. A policy describes how to perform a given task or project.

_____ 10. A personnel manual may also be called an employee handbook.

SHORT ANSWER

1. Describe an organizational chart and its purpose in the medical office.

   _____

   _____

   _____

   _____

   _____

© 2015 Pearson Education, Inc.

2. Describe a mission statement and its purpose in the medical office. Why is it important?

_____

_____

_____

_____

3. Write an example policy for addressing emergencies in the medical office.

_____

_____

_____

_____

4. Write an example policy for addressing staff members being called for jury duty.

_____

_____

_____

_____

5. Write an example policy for addressing requests for vacation time off in the medical office.

_____

_____

_____

_____

6. Write an example policy for addressing staff meetings in the medical office.

_____

_____

_____

_____

7. Write an example policy for addressing sexual harassment in the medical office.

_____

_____

_____

_____

8. Write an example policy for addressing employee evaluations in the medical office.

_____

_____

_____

© 2015 Pearson Education, Inc.   *Office Policies and Procedures*   **135**

9. Write an example policy for addressing absentee issues in the medical office.

_____

_____

_____

_____

10. Write an example policy for addressing patient confidentiality in the medical office.

_____

_____

_____

_____

_____

© 2015 Pearson Education, Inc.

CHAPTER 16

Handling Medical Office Emergencies

CHAPTER OUTLINE

COMPETENCY SKILLS PERFORMANCE

© 2015 Pearson Education, Inc.

CHAPTER REVIEW

- Medical emergencies are rare in the medical office; however, when patients or health care staff become severely ill or injured in the medical office, medical assistants must know how to respond appropriately. Medical assistants play a vital role in medical office emergencies.

- The key to avoiding injuries and accidents in the medical office is to be proactive.

- Medical offices should have well-written and complete policy and procedures manuals that identify the steps to take in the event of a medical office emergency.

- Emergency intervention is called for in any situation that might be life-threatening.

- The medical assistant should be aware of how to handle various medical office emergencies, including fainting (syncope), heart attack, choking, bleeding, shock, fractures, and burns.

- Rescue breathing and CPR are just two means medical staff have to address emergency situations.

- All members of the medical staff, including those who work in the administrative area, should have and maintain current CPR certification as well as knowledge of first aid skills. Instruction in CPR is offered by many medical assisting programs as a separate course. These courses can also be found through the American Red Cross or the American Heart Association (AHA), or through local fire departments or hospitals.

- A number of supplies and equipment help support lifesaving objectives in emergency situations. A crash cart holds a number of supplies and pieces of equipment needed in emergencies.

- The medical assistant should be knowledgeable about emergency preparedness. This includes knowing how to respond in the event of a man-made disaster, such as a terrorist event, or of a natural disaster, such as a hurricane or tornado.

- Mock environmental exposure events may be offered within the community, at colleges, and at hospitals. These events provide real-life scenarios and situations that may take place during a disaster.

LEARNING ACTIVITIES

To ensure that you have achieved the learning objectives in this chapter:

1. In the Terminology Review section on page 139, define the key terminology found in this chapter of your student text.

2. Create a list of community resources that are available either during or after an emergency.

   _____

   _____

   _____

   _____

   _____

APPLIED LEARNING EXERCISES

Using a separate sheet of paper, complete the following assignments:

1. Using an Internet search engine or a local telephone book, write down the contact telephone numbers and corresponding Web sites for each company and organization listed in Learning Activity 2.

2. Create a list of 10 supplies and pieces of equipment that might be found on a crash cart in an ambulatory setting.

© 2015 Pearson Education, Inc.

3. Create a list of emergencies that are not considered life-threatening but do require immediate intervention.

4. Create a list of emergencies that are not life-threatening but require intervention as soon as possible.

5. List the steps to take to assist and monitor a patient who has fainted.

6. Create a list of steps to take to correctly use an automated external defibrillator.

7. Describe the steps to take to stop a patient's nose from bleeding.

8. Write an essay describing the comfort measures that can be taken with patients in various types of emergencies.

TERMINOLOGY REVIEW

Using the glossary and highlighted terms in the textbook, define the following terms:

anaphylaxis: _____

_____

CPR mouth barrier: _____

_____

crash cart: _____

_____

defibrillator: _____

_____

standard precautions: _____

_____

syncope: _____

_____

ABBREVIATIONS

Provide the meanings of the following abbreviations:

AAMA: _____

AED: _____

AHA: _____

CAB: _____

CPR: _____

EECC: _____

EMS: _____

FBOA: _____

FEMA: _____

HEPA: _____

OSHA: _____

PPE: _____

CRITICAL THINKING QUESTIONS

1. Marti Prince, CMA (AAMA), is the office manager in a family practice clinic. She is aware that all members of the medical staff, including those who work in the administrative area, should have and maintain current CPR skills as well as knowledge of first aid skills. What resources might Marti provide those staff members who need to maintain their current CPR certification?

    _____

    _____

    _____

    _____

    _____

2. Al Dobson is taking medical assisting courses at his local community college. He has been given the assignment to write a brief essay on how employees in a health care setting can prevent accidents and injuries. What information might Al include?

    _____

    _____

    _____

    _____

    _____

3. Molly Vitalli, RMA (AMT), is working in an otolaryngology practice. She has been asked by the office manager to create a list of the emergency services telephone numbers that should be kept near the telephone in the medical office. What numbers should Molly include?

    _____

    _____

    _____

    _____

    _____

4. Anne Ogilivie, CMAS (AMT), is the office manager in an OB/GYN clinic. Anne is giving a presentation to her staff about what it means to practice standard precautions in the event the medical assistant may be exposed to blood or other bodily fluids. What information should Anne include?

    _____

    _____

    _____

    _____

    _____

5. Russell Carlson is taking a class on CPR and first aid in the medical office. He has been given an assignment to describe how a CPR mouth barrier is used. What might Russell write?

    _____

    _____

© 2015 Pearson Education, Inc.

_____

_____

_____

_____

CHAPTER REVIEW TEST

MULTIPLE CHOICE

Circle the letter of the correct answer.

1. All of the following materials are needed in order to perform the procedure of adult rescue breathing and cardiopulmonary resuscitation competently EXCEPT _____.
   a. disposable gloves
   b. mouth guard
   c. ventilator mask
   d. approved mannequin
   e. defibrillator

2. Which of the following items is NOT necessary when administering oxygen to a patient?
   a. Portable oxygen tank
   b. Pressure regulator
   c. Stethoscope
   d. Flow meter
   e. Nasal cannula with connecting tubing

3. Which of the following is considered a life-threatening condition?
   a. Extreme shortness of breath
   b. Seizure
   c. Strain
   d. Severe vomiting
   e. Severe diarrhea

4. Which of the following emergency conditions is not considered life-threatening, but does require immediate intervention?
   a. Sprain
   b. Seizure
   c. Cardiac arrest
   d. Head injury
   e. Shock

5. Which of the following conditions is not life-threatening and requires intervention as soon as possible?
   a. Neck injury
   b. Chest pain
   c. Shock
   d. Simple fracture
   e. Head injury

6. CAB stands for _____.
   a. compressions, airway, breathing
   b. compressions, airway, breath sounds
   c. circulation, airway, breathing
   d. circulation, assistance, breathing
   e. compressions, assistance, breathing

7. The most common signs of shock include all of the following EXCEPT _____.

    a. pale, gray, or bluish skin   d. dilated pupils

    b. pain in the biceps   e. extreme thirst

    c. moist, cool skin

8. All of the following are signs of a heart attack EXCEPT _____.

    a. chest pain   d. cold, clammy skin

    b. excessive sweating   e. shortness of breath

    c. extreme thirst

9. In the event of an emergency in the medical setting, which member of the medical staff should be the one to call for emergency services?

    a. The physician   d. The medical assistant

    b. The nurse   e. The physician assistant

    c. The patient

10. An automated external defibrillator is used for what type of emergency?

    a. A patients who has no pulse   d. A patient who has had a seizure

    b. A patient who has sustained a blow to the head   e. A patient who has been poisoned.

    c. A patient with a broken bone

TRUE/FALSE

Identify whether the statement is true (T) or false (F).

_____ 1. Unless the crash cart is used, it does not need to be regularly inventoried.

_____ 2. Staff should rotate supplies kept on the crash cart based on the expiration date.

_____ 3. Every medical office must have a defibrillator for emergency use.

_____ 4. The signs and symptoms of heart attack may differ from one patient to another.

_____ 5. Men and women exhibit the exact same symptoms when experiencing a heart attack.

_____ 6. If a choking patient cannot make any sounds, it is likely that patient's airway is blocked.

_____ 7. The steps to take with a choking infant are the same as the steps to take with a choking adult.

_____ 8. A patient in shock should be covered with a blanket for warmth.

_____ 9. Patients with fractures most likely require emergency room care.

_____ 10. Patients with fractures should be moved only as necessary.

SHORT ANSWER

1. What is anaphylaxis?

_____

_____

_____

 © 2015 Pearson Education, Inc.

2. What is important for the medical assistant to remember with regard to performing within his or her scope of practice during an emergency?

_____

_____

_____

_____

_____

3. When should the medical assistant call emergency services to the medical office?

_____

_____

_____

_____

_____

4. Name five disorders that could cause fainting in a patient.

_____

_____

_____

_____

_____

5. What is Hands-Only CPR?

_____

_____

_____

_____

_____

6. What guidelines should be followed with regard to maintaining emergency supplies in the medical office?

_____

_____

_____

_____

_____

_____

7. Describe how to care for a patient with a fracture.

_____

_____

_____

_____

_____

© 2015 Pearson Education, Inc.

8. How might oxygen be administered to a patient during an emergency?

_____

_____

_____

_____

9. Describe the most common signs and symptoms of a heart attack.

_____

_____

_____

_____

10. What are the signs and symptoms of choking, and how should the medical assistant respond to a patient who is choking?

_____

_____

_____

_____

_____

_____

_____

© 2015 Pearson Education, Inc.

CHAPTER 17
Insurance Billing

CHAPTER OUTLINE

Introduction

Health Insurance Policies

Health Insurance Payers

Health Insurance Claims

Review

COMPETENCY SKILLS PERFORMANCE

Procedure 17-1: Calculate Deductible, Coinsurance, and Allowable Amounts

Procedure 17-2: Verify a Patient's Insurance Eligibility

Procedure 17-3: Obtain a Managed Care Referral

Procedure 17-4: Obtain Authorization from an Insurance Company for a Procedure

Procedure 17-5: Handle a Denied Insurance Claim

Procedure 17-6: Abstract Data to Complete a Paper CMS-1500 Claim Form

Procedure 17-7: Complete a Computerized Insurance Claim Form

CHAPTER REVIEW

- Preparing health insurance forms correctly is vital to the success of any medical practice. Medical offices bill insurance companies and patients to receive payment for their services. They must receive payment in a timely manner in order to hire staff, pay bills, and continue serving patients. Medical assistants play a vital role in this process. They must know how to prepare health insurance claims accurately, follow up on past-due claims, and pursue unpaid amounts.

- Health insurance as it began over 150 years ago bears little resemblance to the modern array of plans and services. Recent federal legislation is expected to change the health insurance landscape further during the next decade.

- Today, Americans obtain health insurance from a variety of sources that are regulated by a multitude of state and federal laws. Medical assistants should have knowledge of the various sources of health insurance, policy provisions and terminology, types of health insurance plans, and types of service coverage.

- In addition to the type of managed care and the type of service coverage, a patient's insurance benefits are also determined by the type of payer. Third-party payers are organizations that pay for health care services on behalf of the patient. In legal terms, the physician is the first party, the patient is the second party, and the payer is the third party.

© 2015 Pearson Education, Inc.

- The federal and state governments provide health insurance for designated groups of people, such as the elderly, the disabled, military personnel and retirees, and injured workers. Each of these programs has its own eligibility requirements and benefit structure. Government insurance includes Medicare, Medicaid, and TRICARE.

- Third-party liability insurance is insurance in which someone other than the patient is ultimately responsible for the medical bills, usually due to injury or negligence. The most common of these types of insurance are workers' compensation insurance and property and casualty insurance.

- Disability income insurance reimburses a patient for lost wages due to a non-work-related disability that prevents the individual from working. The MA's role with disability insurance varies, depending on the role of the physicians in the office.

- There are many steps involved in converting a patient encounter into a paid insurance claim. Each step needs to be completed in a timely and accurate manner in order for providers to receive correct payment for their services.

- The general process for completing an insurance claim is similar from one office to the next. The process begins with the medical assistant gathering accurate patient information. Next, the claims must be prepared and submitted, either electronically or on paper. Finally, payments must be posted, and medical assistants must follow up on unpaid claims to be sure all monies are received.

- Almost all physicians submit insurance claims electronically; however, some smaller offices still use paper forms. Regardless of the submission method used, the same information is required.

- Medical assistants must submit all paper claims using the CMS-1500 claim form. Dental claims are prepared using the American Dental Association (ADA) standard form. Effective April 1, 2014, a new version of the CMS-1500 form is required, due to the implementation of the ICD-10-CM coding system.

- One of the purposes of HIPAA is to standardize how electronic transmissions are handled. Electronic transactions, also called *electronic data interchange* (EDI), are exchanges involving the computerized transfer of health care information between two parties for specific purposes, such as a health care provider submitting medical claims to a health plan for payment. Version 5010 is the set of standards used for all health care transactions.

- Each process that was once handled on paper has a corresponding electronic format. Just as the CMS-1500 form is the standard for paper claims, the 837P is the standard format for electronic claims.

- As a result of the growth of managed care and ongoing concerns about controlling health care costs, insurance companies use a variety of methods to determine how much to pay providers. MAs need to understand how the payment method impacts the practice.

- To post insurance payments, MAs must read and interpret the explanation of benefits, enter data into the computer, and follow up on unpaid claims.

LEARNING ACTIVITIES

To ensure that you have achieved the learning objectives in this chapter:

1. In the Terminology Review section on page 148, define the key terminology found in this chapter of your student text.

2. Create a list of the features of both group and individual health care plans.

_____

_____

_____

_____

© 2015 Pearson Education, Inc.

_____
_____
_____
_____

3. Create a list of the features of PPOs and HMOs.

_____
_____
_____
_____
_____
_____

4. Create a list of the features of government insurance programs.

_____
_____
_____
_____

5. Describe reimbursement methods.

_____
_____
_____
_____

6. Create a list of the steps to follow to prepare an insurance claim.

_____
_____
_____
_____

7. Create a list of the steps to follow for accurate health care claim processing.

_____
_____
_____
_____

8. Create a list of the steps to follow to post insurance payments.

_____
_____
_____

_____

9. Describe the steps to take to trace past-due insurance claims.

_____

_____

_____

_____

10. Create a list of steps for reconciling payments and rejections.

_____

_____

_____

_____

_____

APPLIED LEARNING EXERCISES

Using a separate sheet of paper, complete the following assignments:

1. Write an essay outlining the medical assistant's role in insurance claim processing.
2. Using the Internet, go to Medicare's Web site. Research information on each of the Medicare parts, and write an essay describing Medicare parts A, B, and D coverage.
3. Using the Medicare Web site as a resource, research the criteria for being covered under the Medicare parts A and B plans. Create a list describing the persons who may be covered under Medicare.
4. Using the Internet as a research source, find your state's Medicaid Web site, and research the criteria for being covered under Medicaid in your state. Write an essay describing the persons who may be covered under Medicaid in your state.
5. Using the Internet as a research source, find your state's workers' compensation Web site. Write an essay explaining how to bill for a workers' compensation claim in your state.

TERMINOLOGY REVIEW

Using the glossary and highlighted terms in the textbook, define the following terms:

accept assignment: _____

_____

advance beneficiary notice: _____

_____

allowed amount: _____

_____

appeal: _____

_____

assignment of benefits: _____

_____

                                    © 2015 Pearson Education, Inc.

balance billing: _____

_____

beneficiary: _____

_____

birthday rule: _____

_____

bundle: _____

_____

capitation: _____

_____

certificate of coverage: _____

_____

CHAMPVA: _____

_____

clean claim: _____

_____

closed panel: _____

_____

coinsurance: _____

_____

conversion factor: _____

_____

coordination of benefits: _____

_____

copayment: _____

_____

covered: _____

_____

deductible: _____

_____

denied: _____

_____

dependent: _____

_____

disability income insurance: _____

_____

elective procedure: _____

_____

eligibility: _____

_____

encounter form: _____

exclusions: _____

exclusive provider organization: _____

explanation of benefits: _____

fee-for-service: _____

fee schedule: _____

First Report of Injury or Illness: _____

geographic adjustment factor: _____

group health insurance: _____

health insurance exchange: _____

health maintenance organization: _____

individual health insurance: _____

individual mandate: _____

insured: _____

Item: _____

liability insurance: _____

lifetime maximum benefit: _____

long-term disability: _____

managed care organization: _____

Medicaid: _____

© 2015 Pearson Education, Inc.

medical necessity: _____

Medicare: _____

Medicare Severity-Adjusted Diagnosis-Related Groups: _____

Medigap: _____

member: _____

negotiated fee schedule: _____

non-covered: _____

open-panel: _____

outliers: _____

participating provider: _____

Patient Protection and Affordable Care Act: _____

personal injury protection: _____

point of service: _____

policyholder: _____

preauthorization: _____

pre-existing condition: _____

preferred provider organization: _____

premium: _____

preventive care: _____

primary care provider: _____

private health insurance: _____

_____

progress report: _____

_____

property and casualty insurance: _____

_____

rejected: _____

_____

relative value unit: _____

_____

self-funded: _____

_____

short-term disability: _____

_____

skilled nursing facility: _____

_____

sliding fee scale: _____

_____

Social Security Disability Insurance: _____

_____

Supplemental Security Income: _____

_____

stop loss: _____

_____

subscriber: _____

_____

third-party administrator: _____

_____

third-party payer: _____

_____

TRICARE: _____

_____

unbundling: _____

_____

usual, customary, and reasonable: _____

_____

waiting period: _____

_____

workers' compensation: _____

_____

© 2015 Pearson Education, Inc.

ABBREVIATIONS

Provide the meanings of the following abbreviations:

ABN: _____

ACA: _____

ADA: _____

BC: _____

BCBSA: _____

BS: _____

CF: _____

CHAMPVA: _____

CHIP: _____

CMS: _____

COB: _____

CPT: _____

DEERS: _____

DI: _____

DME: _____

EOB: _____

EPO: _____

FFS: _____

GAF: _____

GHI: _____

HIE: _____

HIPAA: _____

HMO: _____

ICD-10-CM: _____

LTD: _____

MAC: _____

MCO: _____

MCD: _____

MCR: _____

MG: _____

MPFS: _____

MS-DRG: _____

MSP: _____

Non-PAR: _____

NPI: _____

NUCC: _____

OCR: _____

OHI: _____

PAR: _____

P/C: _____

© 2015 Pearson Education, Inc.

PCP: _____

PIP: _____

POS: _____

PPACA: _____

PPO: _____

RBRVS: _____

RVU: _____

SNF: _____

SSDI: _____

SSI: _____

STD: _____

TPA: _____

UCR: _____

WC: _____

CRITICAL THINKING QUESTIONS

1. Josie Svien, CMA (AAMA), is working in the billing office of a family practice clinic. Josie is having trouble reading the handwritten chart notes of one of the clinic physicians. How should Josie proceed with billing for the services in this patient's chart?

   _____

   _____

   _____

   _____

   _____

2. Sean Quinn, RMA (AMT), has been hired to work in the billing office of a large general surgery practice. Sean has been asked to go through several outstanding insurance claims and determine why they have not been paid. As Sean looks through the files, he discovers that many of the claims have never been billed to the insurance carrier. Some of the claims are over a year old, and Sean realizes those may be considered past timely filing limits. What can Sean do in this situation?

   _____

   _____

   _____

   _____

   _____

3. Monica Swinger is taking an administrative medical assisting course. She has been given the assignment to write an essay describing how health insurance began in the United States. What information should Monica include?

   _____

   _____

© 2015 Pearson Education, Inc.

_____

_____

_____

_____

4. Erica Owsley, CMA (AAMA), is working with Charles Wong, a patient in the clinic where Erica works. Mr. Wong tells Erica he has the option of buying into the group insurance plan his employer offers or he can buy an individual policy on his own. He isn't sure which option to choose and asks Erica if she can tell him the difference between individual and group insurance plans. What can Erica tell Mr. Wong?

_____

_____

_____

_____

_____

5. Abraham Long is a patient of Dr. Roland who has recently gotten married; his wife has two children from a previous marriage. He tells Dr. Roland's medical assistant that both he and his new wife have insurance coverage, and he wants to know how to determine which insurance plan will be primary and which will be secondary for his stepchildren. What can the medical assistant tell Mr. Long?

_____

_____

_____

_____

_____

CHAPTER REVIEW TEST

MULTIPLE CHOICE

Circle the letter of the correct answer.

1. _____ is (are) an emergency safety net to protect against unexpected, high-cost medical services only.

   a. Preventive care
   b. Holistic care
   c. Chronic care
   d. Catastrophic care
   e. Ancillary services

2. _____ is care a patient receives to stay well.

   a. Preventive care
   b. Holistic care
   c. Chronic care
   d. Catastrophic care
   e. Disease-specific care

3. An example of preventive care is _____.
   a. a well-child check
   b. treatment for a burn
   c. antibiotics for an infection
   d. a yearly mammogram
   e. All of the above

4. The person who owns the insurance policy is known as the _____.
   a. member
   b. subscriber
   c. insured
   d. policyholder
   e. All of the above

5. In an employer-sponsored health care plan, who pays for the insurance premium?
   a. The employer
   b. The employee
   c. The employer and the employee
   d. The government
   e. The insurance company

6. Which of the following is typically the most expensive type of insurance plan to purchase?
   a. Medicare Part A
   b. Group insurance
   c. Individual insurance
   d. Medicaid
   e. Medicare Part D

7. Which of the following types of insurance plan is least common today?
   a. Fee-for-service plans
   b. Consumer-directed insurance plans
   c. Medicare
   d. Medicaid
   e. Health insurance exchanges

8. Which of the following insurance plans does not typically have a list of physicians the patient is allowed to see in order to obtain the highest level of reimbursement?
   a. Medicaid
   b. Fee-for-service plans
   c. HMO
   d. PPO
   e. Medicare

9. Health care providers who sign contracts to participate with a managed care organization are called _____.
   a. performing providers
   b. participating providers
   c. health care associates
   d. managed care providers
   e. None of the above

10. _____ are any conditions patients were diagnosed with or treated for before beginning coverage with a new insurance plan.
    a. Pre-existing conditions
    b. Catastrophic conditions
    c. Preventive conditions
    d. Progressive conditions
    e. None of the above

TRUE/FALSE

Identify whether the statement is true (T) or false (F).

_____ 1. Every state has a Children's Health Insurance Program (CHIP).

_____ 2. Third-party liability insurance is insurance in which the patient is ultimately responsible for the medical bills.

 © 2015 Pearson Education, Inc.

_____ 3. CHAMPVA covers the health care expenses of retired veterans.

_____ 4. Most patients are well aware of what their insurance covers.

_____ 5. Capitation is a reimbursement method in which providers are paid set fees per month per member patients.

_____ 6. An exclusive provider organization is a group of physicians or medical centers that provides comprehensive service to members under a capitated payment plan.

_____ 7. A health maintenance organization is a company that attempts to control the cost of health care while providing better outcomes by transferring financial risk to the provider.

_____ 8. A sliding fee scale is a provider's fee schedule that charges varying fees for a service based on a patient's financial ability to pay.

_____ 9. Medicaid is a federal program that covers medical expenses for those aged 65 and over, those with end-stage renal disease, and those with long-term disabilities.

_____ 10. Preauthorization is approval for treatment or service obtained from an insurance company before the care is provided.

SHORT ANSWER

1. Explain how workers' compensation insurance coverage works.

_____
_____
_____
_____
_____

2. Describe how a deductible is calculated.

_____
_____
_____
_____
_____

3. Define copayments and coinsurance.

_____
_____
_____
_____
_____

4. Describe what is meant by an insurance company's "approved" or "allowed" amount.

_____
_____
_____
_____
_____

5. What is medical necessity?

_____

_____

_____

_____

_____

6. Define balance billing.

_____

_____

_____

_____

_____

7. What does it mean when a patient signs an assignment of benefits form? What is the benefit to the provider?

_____

_____

_____

_____

_____

8. What is by a pre-existing condition? Are health insurance companies allowed to charge more to individuals with pre-existing conditions?

_____

_____

_____

_____

_____

9. What qualifications must a patient have to be covered under Medicare?

_____

_____

_____

_____

10. What does COBRA require of employers?

_____

_____

_____

_____

_____

© 2015 Pearson Education, Inc.

Diagnostic Coding

CHAPTER OUTLINE

COMPETENCY SKILLS PERFORMANCE

Procedure 18-1: Perform Diagnostic Coding using ICD-10-CM

CHAPTER REVIEW

- Diagnostic coding is the process of assigning a number to a description of the patient's condition, illness, disease, or other reason for the encounter as it appears in the health care provider's documentation in the patient's record.

- Diagnostic codes identify the reasons that health care services were provided.

- ICD-10-CM is a listing of alphanumeric codes, three to seven characters long, and descriptions used to report causes of mortality and morbidity.

- Diagnostic coding has existed for more than a century, beginning with French physician, Jacques Bertillon, who created the Bertillon Classification of Causes of Death.

- A series of delays has repeatedly postponed the ICD-10-CM implementation date. Refer to www.cms.gov for information on the current status of ICD-10-CM.

- The implementation of ICD-10-CM is one of health care's top priorities and expenditures for the next several years because it will take several years after the implementation date for providers and payers to fully adjust to the new system.

- Medical assistants usually do not perform medical coding as a regular part of their job because most medical offices hire or contract with professional certified coders who are trained in the details of assigning medical codes. However, the need occasionally arises for MAs to research a code.

- The ICD-10-CM manual provides the codes that identify all diagnoses physicians give patients.

- Medical assistants abstract information from the medical record in order to code for services and the reasons they were provided. Coding must be performed to the highest level of certainty. All relevant information should be coded, but missing information should never be assumed or coded.

© 2015 Pearson Education, Inc.

- Diagnosis coding involves three basic steps: (1) Identify the first-listed diagnosis; (2) research the diagnosis code in the Index; (3) verify the code(s) in the Tabular List.
- A number of conditions and circumstances in diagnosis coding have unique tables, codes, and guidelines.
- Medical assistants may choose to pursue certification as a professional coder. The Certified Professional Coder (CPC) credential is offered by the AAPC, and the Certified Coding Specialist-Physician based (CCS-P) is offered by AHIMA.

LEARNING ACTIVITIES

To ensure that you have achieved the learning objectives in this chapter:

1. In the Terminology Review section below, define the key terminology found in this chapter of your student text.
2. Create a list of the steps to follow to correctly choose a diagnosis code.

_____

_____

_____

_____

_____

_____

APPLIED LEARNING EXERCISES

Using an ICD-10-CM coding manual, find the correct diagnosis codes for the following conditions:

1. Type I diabetes with ketoacidosis: ICD-10-CM Code(s): _____
2. Acute idiopathic pericarditis: ICD-10-CM Code(s): _____
3. Acute lymphadenitis: ICD-10-CM Code(s): _____
4. Pneumococcal meningitis: ICD-10-CM Code(s): _____

TERMINOLOGY REVIEW

Using the glossary and highlighted terms in the textbook, define the following terms:

category: _____

_____

chapter: _____

_____

chief complaint: _____

_____

code: _____

_____

© 2015 Pearson Education, Inc.

combination code: _____

_____

conventions: _____

_____

etiology: _____

_____

first-listed: _____

_____

Index to Diseases and Injuries: _____

_____

Main Term (ICD-10-CM): _____

_____

morbidity: _____

_____

mortality: _____

_____

multiple coding: _____

_____

neoplasm: _____

_____

nonessential modifiers: _____

_____

primary diagnosis: _____

_____

qualified: _____

_____

secondary diagnoses: _____

_____

section: _____

_____

sequela: _____

_____

sign: _____

_____

subcategory: _____

_____

subterm: _____

_____

symptom: _____

_____

Tabular List (ICD-10-CM): _____

_____

verify: _____

_____

ABBREVIATIONS

Provide the meanings of the following abbreviations:

AAPC: _____

AHIMA: _____

CCS-P: _____

CPC: _____

ICD-9-CM: _____

ICD-10-CM: _____

CRITICAL THINKING QUESTIONS

1. Teresa Clymer, RMA (AMT), is the office manager at the Pine Plains Medical Center. She is preparing her office staff for the implementation of ICD-10-CM. Some staff members are anxious about the transition from ICD-9 to ICD-10. How might Teresa explain to her staff the impact of this transition on the health care system?

   _____

   _____

   _____

   _____

   _____

   _____

2. Anthony Fabiano, CMA (AAMA), is the administrative medical assistant at the Pine Plains Medical Center. He has been asked to code the following patient scenario:

   A patient presents to the medical office complaining of a headache and sore throat. The physician orders a throat culture to check for strep throat.

   Why must Anthony ensure that the claim form carries a diagnostic code that relates to the sore throat?

   _____

   _____

   _____

   _____

   _____

   _____

© 2015 Pearson Education, Inc.

3. Benjamin Tho, CMA (AAMA), is responsible for insurance billing and coding at the Westchester Family Practice. A patient presents to the office complaining of chest pain. The physician believes the pain is symptomatic of heartburn and treats the patient for heartburn. If Benjamin were to code for acute myocardial infarction because he viewed the term *chest pain* in the medical record, how might this incorrect diagnosis coding impact the patient?

_____

_____

_____

_____

_____

4. Marc Alaimo, CMAS (AMT), is a new administrative medical assistant at the West View Medical Center. He is coding services for patients seen during the past week and needs to determine which ICD-10-CM coding manual to use. How might the medical office manager advise Marc?

_____

_____

_____

_____

_____

5. Amanda Forester, RMA (AMT), is the medical office manager at the Westchester Medical Clinic. She has planned to outsource the medical facility's billing to a company that provides such services. What must Amanda take into consideration when working with this company?

_____

_____

_____

_____

_____

CHAPTER REVIEW TEST

MULTIPLE CHOICE

Circle the letter of the correct answer.

1. Diagnostic coding has existed since what year?

   a. 1793
   b. 1893
   c. 1993
   d. 2003
   e. 2014

2. _____ is a listing of alphanumeric codes, three to seven characters long, and descriptions used to report causes of morbidity and mortality.

   a. CPT®
   b. ICD-9-CM
   c. ICD-10-CM
   d. HCPCS
   e. ICD-1

3. Medical offices report diagnosis codes on _____ forms to justify the reasons that services were provided.

   a. patient history
   b. patient registration
   c. HIPAA compliance
   d. CMS-1500
   e. UB-04

4. ICD-10-CM contains _____ codes.

   a. 70,000+
   b. 16,000+
   c. 42,000+
   d. 20,000+
   e. 168,000+

5. What is the code length of ICD-10-CM codes?

   a. 5–8 characters
   b. 3–7 characters
   c. 8–9 characters
   d. 3 characters
   e. 10 characters

6. All of the following are true of ICD-10-CM codes EXCEPT:

   a. There are 70,000+ codes.
   b. The 4th, 5th, and 6th characters are for etiology, anatomic site, and severity.
   c. The second character is always numeric.
   d. The first character is always numeric.
   e. A decimal point is mandatory after the 3rd character on all codes.

7. _____ in the ICD-10-CM manual is an alphabetical list of diseases and injuries, reasons for encounters, and external causes.

   a. The Index
   b. The Tabular List
   c. The Alphabetic Index
   d. The Introductory Material
   e. Appendix A

8. _____ in the ICD-10-CM manual is the alphanumeric list of diseases and injuries, reasons for encounters, and external causes.

   a. The Index
   b. The Tabular List
   c. The Alphabetic Index
   d. The Introductory Material
   e. Appendix A

9. ICD-10-CM conventions are found in _____ of the ICD-10-CM manual.

   a. the Index
   b. the Tabular List
   c. the Alphabetic Index
   d. the Introductory Material
   e. Appendix A

10. Which of the following appear immediately under a code or heading in the Tabular List?

   a. Excludes1 notes
   b. Excludes2 notes
   c. Combination codes
   d. Modifiers
   e. Placeholders

© 2015 Pearson Education, Inc.

TRUE/FALSE

Identify whether the statement is true (T) or false (F).

_____ 1. A placeholder is a filler character that has no meaning by itself.

_____ 2. The first character of an ICD-10-CM code is reserved for special use, most commonly the episode of care for injuries.

_____ 3. Publishers of the ICD-10-CM manual may use color coding and special symbols to alert users to important information.

_____ 4. The Tabular List is an alphanumerically sequenced list of all diagnosis codes, divided into 21 chapters based on cause, or etiology, and body system.

_____ 5. Coding begins and ends with the patient's CMS-1500 form.

_____ 6. If the medical record is incomplete or inaccurate, it should be corrected or amended before attempting to code.

_____ 7. ICD-10-CM Official Guidelines for Coding and Reporting are located in the Index in the ICD-10-CM manual.

_____ 8. The Tabular List is an alphabetical list of diseases and injuries, reasons for encounters, and external causes.

_____ 9. The Index is a numerical list of diseases and injuries, reasons for encounters, and external causes.

_____ 10. The primary diagnosis is the diagnosis that is chiefly responsible for the outpatient services provided.

SHORT ANSWER

1. What are secondary diagnoses?

_____

_____

_____

_____

_____

2. Explain what is meant by the etiology of a disease or injury.

_____

_____

_____

_____

3. List and describe the three additional references in ICD-10-CM that are used for specialized purposes.

_____

_____

_____

_____

_____

4. Explain the use of nonessential modifiers in coding.

5. What are subterms? Provide two examples.

6. Describe the use of the seventh character of an ICD-10-CM code.

7. What do codes of the highest level of specificity provide?

8. Explain what "conventions" are, and list the two conventions that are most important for the medical assistant.

9. How might the medical assistant pursue certification as a professional coder?

© 2015 Pearson Education, Inc.

10. What is the difference between morbidity and mortality?

_____

_____

_____

_____

_____

© 2015 Pearson Education, Inc.

Procedural Coding

CHAPTER OUTLINE

COMPETENCY SKILLS PERFORMANCE

Procedure 19-1: Code for a Procedure

CHAPTER REVIEW

- Procedural coding is the act of assigning a code to a patient's procedure or service. Procedural codes have been standardized since 1996 and render coding more efficient and accurate.

- Current Procedural Terminology (CPT), Fourth Edition (CPT-4), is a listing of five-character alphanumeric codes and descriptions used to report outpatient medical services and procedures.

- The Health Insurance Portability and Accountability Act (HIPAA) mandates the use of CPT for all covered entities that handle electronic claims related to health care services.

- Today, the CPT manual covers all procedures approved by the Food and Drug Administration (FDA). The CPT lists over 8,800 procedural codes. The CPT manual is updated every year, with changes taking effect January 1 when a new manual is published. Code changes are published by the AMA in conjunction with CMS.

- Procedure codes identify billable services provided to patients. Medical offices report CPT procedure codes on CMS-1500 forms and electronic claims to identify the services provided and the cost of those services.

- Accuracy in coding is important in order to prevent fraud or abuse. Fraud is the act of intentionally billing for services that were never given, including upcoding. Abuse is improper behavior and billing practices that result in improper financial gain but are not fraudulent.

- Procedure coding consists of three basic steps: (1) Abstract the procedure(s) from the patient's medical record; (2) look up the procedure(s) in the Index; (3) select and verify the code in the Tabular List.

CPT is a registered trademark of the American Medical Association.

 © 2015 Pearson Education, Inc.

- Evaluation and Management (E&M) codes describe patient encounters with a physician for the evaluation and management of a health problem.
- The Healthcare Common Procedure Coding System (HCPCS) provides codes for reporting nonphysician services, supplies, or durable medical equipment.
- In order to receive proper payment for medical services, physicians' offices must keep adequate, accurate, and complete patient medical and billing records.
- Proper coding begins with the right tools: an up-to-date CPT coding manual, a HCPCS manual, and a medical dictionary.

LEARNING ACTIVITIES

To ensure that you have achieved the learning objectives in this chapter:

1. In the Terminology Review section on page 170, define the key terminology found in this chapter of your student text.
2. Create a list of the steps to take to abstract procedures from a patient's medical record.

_____
_____
_____
_____
_____
_____

APPLIED LEARNING EXERCISES

Using a separate sheet of paper, complete the following assignments:

1. Using a CPT manual, write a brief essay describing the layout of the CPT coding book.
2. Write a brief essay that discusses how modifiers are used in procedural coding. Give examples of three situations where modifiers should be used.
3. Using the Internet as a research source, go to the Web site for your state's Department of Health. Research the laws that apply to billing for medical services in your state. Create a list of the laws you find relating to fraudulent practices for billing and coding.
4. Match the CPT symbol with the correct meaning.
   1. Moderate sedation is bundled in the code description
   2. FDA approval pending
   3. New code in this edition of the CPT manual
   4. Revised code. The code number is the same but the descriptor has been updated.
   5. Resequenced code
   6. Contains new or revised text.
   7. Enclose synonyms, eponyms, or supplementary descriptors for clarity
   8. Modifier 51 exempt
   9. Add-on code must be used in conjunction with another CPT code.

   a. ⊙
   b. +
   c. ( )
   d. ⊘
   e. ●

f. ▲
g. ►◄
h. #
i. ⊘

TERMINOLOGY REVIEW

Using the glossary and highlighted terms in the textbook, define the following terms:

abuse: _____

_____

add-on code: _____

_____

audit: _____

_____

bilateral: _____

_____

bundling: _____

_____

category (CPT): _____

_____

Category I codes: _____

_____

Category II codes: _____

_____

Category III codes: _____

_____

common descriptor: _____

_____

contributing factors: _____

_____

coordination of care: _____

_____

counseling: _____

_____

Current Procedural Terminology: _____

_____

downcode: _____

_____

edit: _____

_____

established patient: _____

_____

© 2015 Pearson Education, Inc.

Evaluation and Management: _____

examination: _____

face-to-face time: _____

fraud: _____

global period: _____

guidelines: _____

Healthcare Common Procedure Coding System: _____

history: _____

indented code: _____

Index (CPT): _____

inpatient: _____

instructional notes: _____

key component: _____

Level I codes: _____

Level II codes: _____

Level III codes: _____

Main Term (CPT): _____

medical decision making: _____

modifier: _____

modifying term: _____

new patient: _____

outpatient: _____

panel: _____

_____

parent code: _____

_____

patient status: _____

_____

presenting problem: _____

_____

procedural coding: _____

_____

procedures: _____

_____

professional component: _____

_____

relative value unit: _____

_____

resequenced code: _____

_____

section: _____

_____

semicolon: _____

_____

special instructions: _____

_____

standalone code: _____

_____

standardized: _____

_____

subcategory: _____

_____

subheading: _____

_____

subsection: _____

_____

surgical package: _____

_____

Tabular List: _____

_____

technical component: _____

_____

unbundling: _____

_____

upcode: _____

_____

© 2015 Pearson Education, Inc.

ABBREVIATIONS

Provide the meanings of the following abbreviations:

AMA: _____

CMS: _____

CPT: _____

DME: _____

E&M: _____

E/EX: _____

FDA: _____

H/HX: _____

HCPCS: _____

MDM: _____

POS: _____

RVU: _____

CRITICAL THINKING QUESTIONS

1. Henry Bagualin, RMA (AMT), is the administrative medical assistant in Dr. Kleinhold's office. Janice Anderson is a patient of Dr. Kleinhold's, and she recently received sutures for a wound. Henry is reviewing her medical record and must assign the correct code for the patient's sutures. In this case, why is it very important that Henry understand the nuances among codes that might be similar?

   _____

   _____

   _____

   _____

   _____

2. Kira Stansfield, CMA (AAMA), is working with Dr. Ramey in an internal medicine clinic. Dr. Ramey is unsure which Evaluation and Management code to choose for certain patients she has seen. How can Kira advise Dr. Ramey in choosing the appropriate code?

   _____

   _____

   _____

   _____

   _____

3. Joyce Shawger is taking an administrative medical assisting course. She has been given the assignment of listing the key components within each subcategory that are used for E&M code selection. What should Joyce include in her list?

   _____

   _____

   _____

_____

_____

_____

4. Gloria Heritage, RMA (AMT), is working in the billing office of a pediatric practice. One of the physicians in the practice frequently chooses a high level E&M code when billing for his patients. When Gloria consults the patient's charts, she finds that there is not sufficient information to use the higher billing codes and determines a lower code would be more appropriate. What can Gloria do in this situation?

_____

_____

_____

_____

_____

5. James Douglas, CMA (AAMA), is working for Dr. Boyan. James notices that Dr. Boyan frequently forgets to chart every detail about his patients' visit. Often, Dr. Boyan circles a procedure code for something he hasn't completely charted in the patient's chart. James is concerned that Dr. Boyan will be accused of fraudulent billing practices in the event an insurance company requests copies of a patient's medical chart. How can James address this situation?

_____

_____

_____

_____

_____

CHAPTER REVIEW TEST

MULTIPLE CHOICE

Circle the letter of the correct answer.

1. Procedure codes have been standardized since _____.
   a. 1946
   b. 1956
   c. 1966
   d. 1976
   e. 2013

2. _____ is a listing of five-character alphanumeric codes and descriptions used to report outpatient medical services and procedures.
   a. ICD-9-CM
   b. CPT
   c. E&M
   d. HCPCS
   e. ICD-10-CM

© 2015 Pearson Education, Inc.

3. _____ codes comprise the bulk of the CPT.
   a. Category I
   b. Category II
   c. Category III
   d. E&M
   e. HCPCS

4. _____ codes are temporary codes for data collection and tracking the use of emerging technology, services, and procedures.
   a. Category I
   b. Category II
   c. Category III
   d. E&M
   e. HCPCS

5. The code set used to code procedures and services in the outpatient health care setting is _____.
   a. CPT
   b. E&M
   c. ICD-9-CM
   d. ICD-10-CM
   e. HCPCS

6. _____ codes are CPT codes that are used for billing physician services to evaluate and manage patient care, such as office visits.
   a. E&M
   b. HCPCS
   c. Level II
   d. Category III
   e. Category V

7. A(n) _____ code is a CPT code that appears out of numerical sequence within a subsection in order to group it with similar codes.
   a. unbundled
   b. standalone
   c. parent
   d. resequenced
   e. HCPCS

8. In the CPT manual, the _____ code is left-justified and begins with a capital letter.
   a. unbundled
   b. resequenced
   c. standalone
   d. indented
   e. bundled

9. The Tabular List contains six sections, which include all of the following EXCEPT _____.
   a. subsections
   b. subcategories
   c. categories
   d. subheadings
   e. appendices

10. When physicians perform procedures that are not listed in the CPT coding book, what must the medical assistant do?
   a. Choose a code for the closest procedure to what was done.
   b. Not bill for the service.
   c. Ask the physician to choose an appropriate code.
   d. Use an unlisted procedure code and submit copies of the procedure report with the claim.
   e. Inform the patient.

TRUE/FALSE

Identify whether the statement is true (T) or false (F).

_____ 1. CPT guidelines are specific instructions at the beginning of each section of the CPT manual that define terms and describe specific information about how to use codes in that section.

_____ 2. Medical decision making is a key component of E&M coding that describes the complexity of establishing a diagnosis and/or selecting a management option.

_____ 3. A modifier is a three-character alphanumeric code appended to CPT or Level II codes to further describe circumstances.

_____ 4. Category II codes comprise the bulk of the CPT manual.

_____ 5. E&M codes are the most frequently used and are used by all medical specialties.

_____ 6. Modifying terms are descriptive words in the Index that appear indented under the Main Term to further describe the service or procedure.

_____ 7. HPCPS codes describe patient encounters with a physician for the evaluation and management of a health problem.

_____ 8. Evaluation and Management codes are a set of codes developed and maintained by CMS for reporting of professional services, nonphysician services, supplies, durable medical equipment, and injectable drugs.

_____ 9. Medical assistants may work in offices that use certified coders to assign and audit procedure codes.

_____ 10. On the CMS-1500 form, each CPT code must be cross-referenced to one or more diagnosis codes that identify the medical reason each service was provided.

SHORT ANSWER

1. What might be the consequences of reporting incorrect procedure codes on an insurance claim?

_____

_____

_____

_____

_____

2. Examination (E/EX) describes the complexity of the physical assessment of the patient. How is complexity classified?

_____

_____

_____

_____

_____

© 2015 Pearson Education, Inc.

3. What are the four types of medical decision making?

_____

_____

_____

_____

_____

4. What do Category I codes describe?

_____

_____

_____

_____

5. What are Category II codes?

_____

_____

_____

_____

6. Describe the Index in the CPT manual.

_____

_____

_____

_____

7. Describe the role of the medical assistant in coding.

_____

_____

_____

_____

8. How do medical offices report procedure codes?

_____

_____

_____

_____

9. What is meant by the "professional component" of a test or procedure?

_____

_____

_____

10. What is included in the CPT surgical package?

_____

_____

_____

_____

_____

© 2015 Pearson Education, Inc.

CHAPTER 20

Billing, Collections, and Credit

CHAPTER OUTLINE

COMPETENCY SKILLS PERFORMANCE

CHAPTER REVIEW

- The best computerized medical systems for billing, collections, and credit are those that include software that is both functional and useful in tracking accounts and payments, as well as advanced features that support the medical facility's business objectives.

- Professional fees are determined by a set of defined criteria so medical offices can operate within a fair and consistent fee schedule.

- The medical office's accounts receivable are the accounts that are owed by patients for services rendered. It is very important for the medical assistant to keep track of and remain consistent with the accounts receivables in the medical office.

- When accounts are no longer considered collectable by the medical office, the account may be turned over to a collection agency or taken to small claims court. Collection agencies should be fair and equitable while being effective.

- Occasionally, out of professional courtesy, physicians may treat patients they know personally without charging the patient for the service, or for a reduced fee.

- When patients are unable to afford the cost of services, the physician may choose to give the patient a hardship discount. In order to do this, specific steps must be followed. When otherwise able patients fail to honor their financial obligations, small claims courts can help medical offices collect their past-due accounts.

LEARNING ACTIVITIES

To ensure that you have achieved the learning objectives in this chapter:

1. In the Terminology Review section on page 181, define the key terminology found in this chapter of your student text.

2. Create a list of the desired features in a computerized medical billing system.

_____

_____

_____

_____

3. Create a list of the steps to take to post a nonsufficient funds check.

_____

_____

_____

_____

_____

_____

_____

4. Create a list of steps to take to review a managed care contract. Include a list of the pros and cons for a health care provider to sign managed care contracts.

_____

_____

_____

_____

_____

_____

_____

© 2015 Pearson Education, Inc.

5. Create a list of initial steps to take to collect money on past-due accounts.

_____
_____
_____
_____
_____
_____
_____
_____
_____
_____
_____

APPLIED LEARNING EXERCISES

Using a separate sheet of paper, complete the following assignments:

1. Call a local medical office in your area, introduce yourself as a student, and ask to speak to someone in the billing office. Ask this person if you may conduct an interview about his or her job function. Ask the individual the following questions:
   - What type of system does this office use for billing (manual or computerized)?
   - If the office uses a computer system for billing, what is the name of the software used?
   - What functions does the computer system have that help the billing office staff better perform their jobs?
2. Write an essay outlining how professional fees are determined.
3. Write a sample office policy for collecting payments from patients in the medical office.
4. Using the Internet as a research source, look up three collection agencies that offer their services in your area. List the pros and cons for using these three companies.
5. Write a brief essay explaining how professional courtesy applies in the medical office.
6. Write a brief essay describing how hardship discounts are used in the medical office.
7. Using the Internet as a research source, look up the laws regarding the use of small claims court in your state. Write a 1–2 page essay explaining how small claims court may be used to collect overdue accounts in a medical office in your state.

TERMINOLOGY REVIEW

Using the glossary and highlighted terms in the textbook, define the following terms:

accounts receivables (AR): _____
_____

aging report: _____
_____

certified letter: _____
_____

collection agency: _____
_____

community property laws: _____
_____

dual fee schedule: _____

Fair Debt Collection Practices Act (FDCPA): _____

fee schedule: _____

geographic practice cost index (GPCI): _____

hardship agreement: _____

insurance fraud: _____

national conversion factor: _____

national standard: _____

Omnibus Budget Reconciliation Act (OBRA): _____

patient billing statements: _____

post: _____

professional courtesy: _____

Red Flags Rule: _____

relative value unit (RVU): _____

tickler file: _____

uncollectible: _____

write off: _____

ABBREVIATIONS

Provide the meanings of the following abbreviations:

AR: _____

CMS: _____

CPT: _____

© 2015 Pearson Education, Inc.

FDCPA: _____

GPCI: _____

HIPAA: _____

NSF: _____

OBRA: _____

RBRVS: _____

RVU: _____

CRITICAL THINKING QUESTIONS

1. Marissa Duchenne, CMA (AAMA), has been newly hired as the office manager in a multispecialty clinic. When she goes over the clinic's fee schedule, Marissa finds that the clinic has several different fee levels associated with the same procedure codes. When Marissa questions the office staff, she finds that patients who have no insurance coverage are charged nearly 40 percent less for the same services as patients who have insurance coverage. What can Marissa say to the physicians about this practice?

_____

_____

_____

_____

_____

_____

2. Susan Doerr, CMAA (NHA), is working in the billing office in a small family practice clinic. The physicians are considering the pros and cons of taking credit card payments in the clinic and have asked Susan to research the fees incurred by the medical practice for accepting credit card payments from patients. What can Susan tell the physicians about taking credit card payments?

_____

_____

_____

_____

3. Christopher Hernandez, CMA (AAMA), is working at the front desk of a gastroenterology practice. The office has been having difficulty with patients' personal checks being returned from the bank for nonsufficient funds. What might Christopher suggest to the office manager to help alleviate this problem?

_____

_____

_____

_____

_____

4. Dr. Roger Dominguez operates a single-physician practice. Dr. Dominguez employs one medical assistant, Garrick Sinclair, RMA (AMT). The clinic has been using a manual accounting system for many years, and Dr. Dominguez has asked Garrick to research the benefits of moving to a computerized billing system as opposed to keeping the manual system. What might Garrick list in his report for Dr. Dominguez?

_____

_____

_____

_____

_____

_____

5. Dr. Klein wants to raise his prices for certain services offered to his patients. How might the medical assistant respond to this?

_____

_____

_____

_____

_____

_____

CHAPTER REVIEW TEST

MULTIPLE CHOICE

Circle the letter of the correct answer.

1. _____ are documents that detail the money owed to the medical practice and how long the account has been outstanding.
   a. Accounts payable
   b. Superbills
   c. Aging reports
   d. Fee schedules
   e. Encounter forms

2. Medical billing software programs can print reports such as _____.
   a. patients' birthdays
   b. female patients over the age of 40 who have not had a mammogram in the past year
   c. male patients over the age of 50 who have not had a colonoscopy in the past year
   d. aging reports
   e. All of the above

3. Which of the following is a benefit of using a computerized billing system in the medical office?
   a. Send electronic insurance bills
   b. Print insurance billing forms
   c. Post insurance payments electronically
   d. Print patient billing forms
   e. All of the above

© 2015 Pearson Education, Inc.

4. The Omnibus Budget Reconciliation Act was passed in _____.
   a. 1973
   b. 1989
   c. 1993
   d. 2003
   e. 2013

5. The resource-based relative value scale was designed to _____.
   a. reduce Medicare costs
   b. reduce fraudulent billing
   c. create a fee schedule that can never be raised
   d. increase medical office revenue
   e. None of the above

6. Medicare service fees are calculated based on all of the following factors EXCEPT _____.
   a. service intensity
   b. time needed for the service
   c. the practice's malpractice premiums
   d. the practice's overhead
   e. the amount the physician wishes to charge

7. The geographic practice cost index adjusts physicians' fees according to what criterion?
   a. Where the practice is located within the United States
   b. The type of specialty the physician practices
   c. The amount of the physician's overhead
   d. The number of employees the physician has
   e. The practice's malpractice premiums

8. The relative value unit was devised by _____ as a way for physicians to create a fee schedule for the services they render.
   a. OSHA
   b. COBRA
   c. CMS
   d. TJC
   e. AMA

9. Participating provider agreements for managed care are _____ pages in length.
   a. 10–20
   b. 20–30
   c. 30–40
   d. 40–50
   e. The length varies depending upon the managed care plan.

10. When should fees be discussed with patients?
   a. Before care is rendered
   b. While care is being rendered
   c. After care is rendered
   d. When the patient is hospitalized
   e. When the office decides to take the patient to small claims court

TRUE/FALSE

Identify whether the statement is true (T) or false (F).

_____ 1. The national standard established by the resource-based relative value scale is based on the current diagnosis codes used for patient visits.

_____ 2. Each year, Medicare assigns a national conversion factor that is added to the relative value unit to determine physicians' fees.

© 2015 Pearson Education, Inc.

_____ 3. Most patients with private health insurance are covered by managed care plans.

_____ 4. When health care providers agree to participate in managed care plans, they agree to accept predetermined fee schedules.

_____ 5. When patients make payment agreements for their account balance, the medical assistant should ask the patient to sign a payment contract agreement.

_____ 6. Patients who clearly understand the physician's fees are more likely to pay their bills in a timely manner.

_____ 7. Many medical offices send new patients copies of the office policy for payment information prior to the first visit.

_____ 8. Part of the reason medical offices request that patients provide the names and telephone numbers of employers and emergency contacts is to give the office additional ways to track the patient should the account become past due.

_____ 9. Every state has the same statute of limitations when it comes to collecting patient debts.

_____ 10. Medical offices should predetermine how much they are willing to extend to patients in credit.

SHORT ANSWER

1. Write an example of a payment contract agreement.

_____

_____

_____

_____

2. What is the statute of limitations in your state regarding collecting past-due patient debts?

_____

_____

_____

_____

3. Explain why the medical office should make a copy of all patients' driver's licenses when they begin care in the medical office.

_____

_____

_____

_____

4. What are accounts receivables in the medical office?

_____

_____

_____

_____

© 2015 Pearson Education, Inc.

5. What are the various ways the medical assistant can contact the patient about a past-due balance?

_____

_____

_____

_____

6. What are the dos and don'ts for collection telephone calls?

_____

_____

_____

_____

_____

7. Describe the message you would leave if you are calling a patient about a past-due balance and someone other than the patient answers the telephone.

_____

_____

_____

_____

_____

8. Explain what is meant by forgiving a patient's deductible or copayment.

_____

_____

_____

_____

_____

9. What is a hardship agreement?

_____

_____

_____

_____

10. How should the medical office handle a situation where a patient with a past-due balance files for bankruptcy?

_____

_____

_____

_____

© 2015 Pearson Education, Inc.

CHAPTER 21
Payroll, Accounts Payable, and Banking Procedures

CHAPTER OUTLINE

COMPETENCY SKILLS PERFORMANCE

CHAPTER REVIEW

- Payroll is a critical function in the medical office and involves keeping accurate records on all employees.

- Accounts payable involves the office paying for bills, rent, utilities, and supplies.

- Banking procedures involve balancing the office checking account and filing appropriate quarterly and yearly statements with state and federal agencies.

- Many large medical offices hire outside firms to help them complete their financial procedures. Smaller offices tend to rely on their physicians or office managers for these tasks.

- Both manual and computerized payroll systems are utilized in health care; however, computerized systems tend to offer greater ease and convenience.

- When depositing payments received, checks must be endorsed properly and deposited following documented procedures.

- Most medical offices keep petty cash funds, small amounts of money to fund spur-of-the-moment costs like out-of-stock office supplies or postage. When money is taken from petty cash, receipts or

© 2015 Pearson Education, Inc.

vouchers in the amount paid and the reason for the expenditure should replace the money in the fund. The petty cash fund should be balanced monthly.

- The bank statement should be reconciled on a monthly basis to ensure that the account balance is accurate and free of errors.

LEARNING ACTIVITIES

To ensure that you have achieved the learning objectives in this chapter:

1. In the Terminology Review section on page 190, define the key terminology found in this chapter of your student text.

2. Create a list of the steps to take to calculate an employee's payroll.

_____

_____

_____

_____

_____

_____

_____

_____

_____

3. Create a list of the types of expenses incurred in the medical office.

_____

_____

_____

_____

_____

_____

_____

_____

4. Create a list of the steps to take to account for petty cash.

_____

_____

_____

_____

5. Create a list of the steps to take to create a deposit of the payments collected in the medical office.

_____

_____

_____

_____

_____

_____

_____

_____

_____

_____

6. Create a list of the steps to take to reconcile a monthly bank statement.

_____

_____

_____

_____

_____

_____

_____

_____

_____

_____

APPLIED LEARNING EXERCISES

Using a separate sheet of paper, complete the following assignments:

1. Call a medical office in your area, introduce yourself as a student, and ask to speak with the office manager/clinic director. If given permission, interview this person about the payroll function in the office. Write a 1–2 page essay discussing how the payroll function is handled in this medical office. Include information on whether the payroll is done in the office or if it is outsourced to another agency.
2. Using the Internet as a research source, look up three different software programs that can perform the payroll function. Create a list of the pros and cons of these three programs as well as manual versus computerized payroll systems.
3. Write an essay describing the function of accounts payable in the medical office.
4. Write a short essay about the uses of petty cash in the medical office.

TERMINOLOGY REVIEW

Using the glossary and highlighted terms in the textbook, define the following terms:

auditors: _____

_____

charitable contributions: _____

_____

Circular E: _____

_____

© 2015 Pearson Education, Inc.

deductions: _____

_____

endorsement stamp: _____

_____

Fair Labor Standards Act: _____

_____

Federal Insurance Contributions Act: _____

_____

Federal Unemployment Tax Act: _____

_____

garnish: _____

_____

gross pay: _____

_____

net pay: _____

_____

outsource: _____

_____

overtime: _____

_____

payroll: _____

_____

payroll taxes: _____

_____

personnel file: _____

_____

quarterly payroll reports: _____

_____

security envelope: _____

_____

Social Security Act: _____

_____

time clock: _____

_____

unemployment insurance: _____

_____

W-2 form: _____

_____

W-4 form: _____

_____

wages: _____

_____

withholding allowances: _____

_____

ABBREVIATIONS

Provide the meanings of the following abbreviations:

FICA: _____

FLSA: _____

FUTA: _____

HIPAA: _____

IRS: _____

CRITICAL THINKING QUESTIONS

1. Ronnie Nguyen, CMA (AAMA), is the office manager for Dr. Hyun Kim. Ronnie has been handling the office payroll with a manual system for several years. Dr. Kim has asked Ronnie to research the possibility of buying software for the payroll function. Dr. Kim wants Ronnie to provide her with a list of pros and cons for manual and computerized systems for the payroll function. What should Ronnie include?

_____

_____

_____

_____

_____

2. As part of an assignment for an administrative medical assisting course, Jordyn Hughes has been asked to write an essay describing the history of payroll in the United States. What should Jordyn include in her essay?

_____

_____

_____

_____

_____

_____

_____

_____

_____

_____

© 2015 Pearson Education, Inc.

3. Francie Crook, CMAA (NHA), has been newly hired to work in a busy family practice clinic. When Francie looks at her first paycheck, she notices that tax has been taken out for something called FICA. She asks her office manager to explain what this tax is. How might the office manager explain this tax to Francie?

_____

_____

_____

_____

_____

_____

4. Linnea Wagner is taking an administrative course as part of her medical assistant training. She has been asked to write an essay explaining how an injured worker's medical bills would be taken care of. What might Linnea include in her paper?

_____

_____

_____

_____

_____

_____

5. Mark Jameelah is taking a course in payroll processing. He has been asked to explain the difference between gross pay and net pay. How should Mark explain the difference?

_____

_____

_____

_____

CHAPTER REVIEW TEST

MULTIPLE CHOICE

Circle the letter of the correct answer.

1. Which of the following would be considered deductions on an employee's payroll?
   a. Federal tax withholding
   b. Vacation pay
   c. Overtime pay
   d. Reimbursement for continuing education courses
   e. None of the above

2. Every business must file _____ payroll reports to the IRS that account for all monies withheld as taxes and deposits made to the IRS of those taxes.

   a. weekly
   b. monthly
   c. bi-monthly
   d. quarterly
   e. yearly

3. Which of the following items might be found in an employee's personnel file?

   a. A copy of the employee's driver's license
   b. A copy of the employee's employment application
   c. A copy of the employee's résumé
   d. The employee's credentials
   e. All of the above

4. How often should an employee's personnel file be updated?

   a. Weekly
   b. Monthly
   c. Yearly
   d. As necessary when information changes
   e. At each employee evaluation

5. In lieu of a Social Security card, employees may provide a copy of their valid _____ as a means of identification.

   a. passport
   b. insurance information form
   c. driver's license
   d. malpractice insurance documentation
   e. I-9 form

6. Which IRS form is used to indicate the employee's withholding allowance?

   a. W-2 form
   b. W-3 form
   c. W-4 form
   d. W-9 form
   e. I-9 form

7. How often should employees update their W-4 form?

   a. Monthly
   b. Yearly
   c. Every 5 years
   d. Every 10 years
   e. Whenever withholding information changes

8. How much is typically paid to employees for overtime wages?

   a. Twice the employee's normal rate of pay
   b. 1.5 times the employee's normal rate of pay
   c. Three times the employee's normal rate of pay
   d. 2.5 times the employee's normal rate of pay
   e. None of the above

9. The _____ IRS form is used to calculate the correct amount of federal withholding tax for an employee.

   a. quarterly report
   b. W-2
   c. Circular E
   d. W-9
   e. I-9

10. To ensure timely payroll processing, employees must complete and sign their _____ before their first payroll period.

    a. Circular E
    b. W-2
    c. W-4
    d. W-9
    e. I-9

© 2015 Pearson Education, Inc.

TRUE/FALSE

Identify whether the statement is true (T) or false (F).

_____ 1. All employers who pay employees an hourly wage must use a time clock.

_____ 2. A salaried employee is not eligible for overtime pay, no matter how many hours the employee works in a given pay period.

_____ 3. Disability insurance is mandatory; all employers must offer it to their employees.

_____ 4. As a general rule, the more exemptions claimed on the W-4 form, the lower the amount of federal taxes that will be withheld.

_____ 5. Medicare withholding tax is 1.45 percent of the employee's gross wages.

_____ 6. Workmen's compensation insurance premiums may be paid partly by the employee.

_____ 7. Many computer software programs that handle the payroll function will also print W-2 forms.

_____ 8. W-2 forms must be postmarked by January 31.

_____ 9. An employer does not have to garnish employee wages if the employee asks him or her not to.

_____ 10. Many suppliers who do business with the medical office will offer discounts under certain payment circumstances.

SHORT ANSWER

1. Explain how a time clock is used in calculating employee hours worked.

_____

_____

_____

_____

_____

2. Explain how an employee who is paid on a salaried basis would be paid for overtime pay.

_____

_____

_____

_____

_____

3. Explain how the Circular E IRS booklet is used to calculate payroll.

_____

_____

_____

_____

_____

4. Explain how garnishment of wages works from the employer's perspective.

_____

_____

_____

5. What is important to consider in the maintenance of the checkbook register?

6. What expenditure categories might be found in the medical office's checkbook register?

7. What methods of payment might the medical office receive from patients for services rendered?

8. Why is an endorsement stamp used in the medical office?

9. What items might be paid from the medical office's petty cash fund?

10. What steps are involved in reconciling a bank statement?

© 2015 Pearson Education, Inc.

CHAPTER 22
Managing the Medical Office

CHAPTER OUTLINE

COMPETENCY SKILLS PERFORMANCE

CHAPTER REVIEW

- The effective medical office manager demonstrates a range of high-level skills, including communication and organization skills, and possibly clinical aptitude.
- Effective staff meetings, which are often led by office managers, usually result from planning that includes detailed, accurate agendas.
- In order to attract and retain appropriately trained and able staff members, the medical office must have detailed job descriptions for every position in the office.
- The medical office might advertise for employees in a variety of settings, from conventional newspapers and Web sites to agencies and colleges.
- Office managers must follow legal guidelines with regard to the questions they ask potential employees during the interview process.
- The hiring process should include research into a potential employee's credentials and past job performance.
- The effective management of employees includes clearly written and understood expectations. Organization, equity, and clear communication are essential. Employment policies that outline such issues as the terms for employee discipline or termination are valuable tools in the medical office. These policies are typically presented in the form of a policy manual.
- Employee evaluations are critical to ensure that employees remain fulfilled and productive in their job role. In order to ensure continued high performance, employees should be evaluated on a regular schedule.
- When providing references for an employee, the reference must remain professional and within legal boundaries.
- Quality improvement programs are a necessary component of a well-run office. These programs look for possible solutions to potential safety problems in the medical office.
- Risk management programs look to improve a situation that has been identified as a possible safety risk to patients or employees. Every member of the medical office staff should be involved in looking for ways to improve safety.
- To ensure patient and employee safety, injury incidents must be reported following specific guidelines.
- Medical office staff must dispose of hazardous waste according to federal and local law.
- Personal protective equipment is designed to safeguard those providing patient care.

LEARNING ACTIVITIES

To ensure that you have achieved the learning objectives in this chapter:

1. In the Terminology Review section on page 200, define the key terminology found in this chapter of your student text.
2. Create a list of the characteristics associated with an effective medical office manager. Include notations as to which of these skills you feel you possess and how you might go about acquiring the skills you are not as strong in.

_____

_____

_____

_____

_____

_____

© 2015 Pearson Education, Inc.

_____
_____
_____
_____

3. Create a list of appropriate questions to ask of a potential employee during an interview.

_____
_____
_____
_____
_____
_____
_____
_____
_____

4. List the guidelines the medical office manager should follow with regard to the performance of employee evaluations.

_____
_____
_____
_____
_____
_____
_____
_____
_____

5. List the steps the medical office manager should follow when providing employee references.

_____
_____
_____
_____
_____
_____
_____
_____

6. List possible sentinel events that might be encountered in the medical office.

_____
_____

_____
_____
_____

7. List several examples of protective equipment that is found in the medical office.

_____
_____
_____
_____

APPLIED LEARNING EXERCISES

Using a separate sheet of paper, complete the following assignments:

1. Write a 1–2 page essay describing the different management styles. Include notations as to which of these management styles you feel you are capable of performing.

2. Write a 1–2 page essay outlining how to conduct an effective staff meeting.

3. Write a 1–2 page essay describing the purpose of a job description. List the items that should be included in a job description.

4. Create a sample staff meeting agenda, with the items that might be included.

5. Using the Internet and your local newspaper as a resource, look for the current job listings for medical assistants in your area. Create a list of these jobs, including any required qualifications.

6. Write a sample job placement ad for an administrative medical assistant.

7. Write a brief essay outlining how to conduct an effective interview.

8. Write a sample office policy for the steps to take to check an employee's professional credentials.

9. Create a sample office policy for the steps to take in calling for employee references.

10. Create a sample office policy for disciplining and terminating employees.

11. Write a brief essay explaining why the medical office needs a sexual harassment policy.

12. Write a brief essay describing the reasons why a medical office would need a quality improvement program and a risk management program.

13. Using the Internet, search for The Joint Commission (TJC) Web site. Write a brief essay describing how and why an incident report is to be used in the medical office.

14. Write a brief essay describing the types, and the appropriate disposal of, hazardous waste in the medical office.

15. Write a sample office policy for addressing employee safety in the medical office.

TERMINOLOGY REVIEW

Using the glossary and highlighted terms in the textbook, define the following terms:

adverse outcome: _____

_____

agenda: _____

_____

body language: _____

_____

© 2015 Pearson Education, Inc.

chemical waste: _____

_____

delegate: _____

_____

Employment Assistance Programs: _____

_____

infectious waste: _____

_____

radioactive waste: _____

_____

sentinel event: _____

_____

sexual harassment: _____

_____

solid waste: _____

_____

ABBREVIATIONS

Provide the meanings of the following abbreviations:

ADA: _____

ADEA: _____

EAP: _____

EEOC: _____

MSDS: _____

CRITICAL THINKING QUESTIONS

1. Shannon Nelson, NHA (CMAA), is working as the office manager in a walk-in clinic. How should she address the clinical medical assistant who is excessively tardy?

   _____

   _____

   _____

   _____

   _____

2. Walter Nichols, CMA (AAMA), is the Westfield Medical Clinic's office manager. He is faced with the uncomfortable task of terminating an employee. How should Walter go about this task?

   _____

   _____

   _____

3. Gina Hagen, RMA (AMT), has been asked to create an office policy for how the weekly staff meetings should be conducted. What might Gina include?

_____

_____

_____

_____

_____

4. Bobbie Kilpatrick, RMA (AMT), has been newly hired to work in a small general practice office. On her first day, Bobbie finds out that the office holds staff meetings twice weekly during the lunch hour. Bobbie's coworkers tell her that lunch is not provided and the time spent at the staff meetings is not compensated. The general feeling of the office staff is to dislike these meetings. How might this office change the employees' attitude toward the staff meetings?

_____

_____

_____

_____

_____

5. At the weekly staff meeting, several items that were not on the agenda have been brought up. Julie, the office manager, wants to end the meeting on time. What can she do about the unexpected items that are brought up?

_____

_____

_____

_____

CHAPTER REVIEW TEST

MULTIPLE CHOICE

Circle the letter of the correct answer.

1. The medical office manager must be _____.

   a. well-organized
   b. honest
   c. a good communicator
   d. able to resolve conflict
   e. All of the above

2. For which leadership style does the leader expect and model an excellent work ethic and self-direction?

   a. Pacesetting
   b. Authoritative
   c. Democratic
   d. Coaching
   e. Coercive

© 2015 Pearson Education, Inc.

3. For which leadership style does the leader ask for opinions and/or advice before making decisions?

   a. Pacesetting
   b. Authoritative
   c. Democratic
   d. Coaching
   e. Coercive

4. The _____ leader makes all decisions without seeking input.

   a. pacesetting
   b. authoritative
   c. democratic
   d. autocratic
   e. coercive

5. How should unexpected items that are brought up at a staff meeting be handled?

   a. They should all be addressed at the time they are brought up.
   b. They should be addressed if they cannot wait; otherwise, they should be added to the agenda for the next meeting.
   c. They should be addressed if the person who brought them up won't be able to make the next meeting.
   d. They should be ignored, since they weren't on the agenda for the current meeting.
   e. They should not be addressed, and the employee who brought them up should be disciplined.

6. Which of the following should be included in the staff meeting minutes?

   a. A description of the items discussed
   b. A list of all staff members at the meeting
   c. The date and time the meeting was held
   d. A brief description of each item discussed
   e. All of the above

7. Which of the following is appropriate to discuss at a staff meeting?

   a. Upcoming holiday office closures
   b. Disciplinary problems with individual staff members
   c. Personal problems experienced by individual staff members
   d. Personal problems shared with staff members by patients
   e. Employee terminations

8. Who should record the minutes from the staff meeting?

   a. The person leading the meeting
   b. The physician
   c. The office manager
   d. Someone other than the person leading the meeting
   e. All of the above

9. Who should receive a copy of the staff meeting minutes?

   a. Staff members who were in attendance
   b. Staff members who were not in attendance
   c. All staff members
   d. The physician and the office manager
   e. Patients

10. Whose responsibility is it to determine the staffing needs of the medical office?

   a. The office manager
   b. The physician
   c. Both the office manager and the physician
   d. The entire staff
   e. The patients

© 2015 Pearson Education, Inc.

TRUE/FALSE

Identify whether the statement is true (T) or false (F).

_____ 1. The medical office manager should be able to adopt different leadership styles depending upon the situation.

_____ 2. Staff meetings should always be led by the physician.

_____ 3. The job description may be used to evaluate current employees' performance.

_____ 4. Job descriptions are the same from one office to another.

_____ 5. Medical offices may recruit employees by posting openings with medical assisting programs local to their area.

_____ 6. Résumés with poor grammar or typographical errors may be discarded by office managers.

_____ 7. To remain consistent from one potential employee to another, the office manager may have a preprinted list of questions to ask.

_____ 8. The office manager should take notes when interviewing potential employees.

_____ 9. The Equal Employment Opportunity Commission enforces the laws against discriminating in hiring practices.

_____ 10. When an employer calls the office for a reference on a former employee, the office manager can decide what information to release on a case-by-case basis.

SHORT ANSWER

1. Explain what it means to be able to multitask.

   _____

   _____

2. Explain what it means to delegate tasks to others.

   _____

   _____

3. Describe the following leadership styles: autocratic, democratic, and laissez-faire.

   _____

   _____

   _____

   _____

4. Explain how to lead an effective staff meeting.

   _____

   _____

   _____

   _____

5. What items should be included in a job description?

   _____

   _____

© 2015 Pearson Education, Inc.

_____

_____

_____

6. What should be included in a job description for a front desk receptionist?

_____

_____

_____

_____

7. Describe the following leadership styles: pacesetting, coaching, and coercive.

_____

_____

_____

_____

_____

8. What questions are illegal to ask a potential employee during an employment interview?

_____

_____

_____

_____

_____

9. What is an Employment Assistance Program (EAP)? What resources do EAPs often include?

_____

_____

_____

_____

_____

10. How does the TJC describe a sentinel event?

_____

_____

_____

_____

_____

CHAPTER OUTLINE

CHAPTER REVIEW

- Though any member of the medical office team may be involved with marketing initiatives in the medical office, in offices where there is a dedicated office manager, that person is typically the one leading the marketing efforts.

- A marketing plan is a comprehensive plan that outlines a business's overall marketing objectives in a given period.

- The clinic's marketing budget is the amount of money allocated to promote the clinic's products or services.

© 2015 Pearson Education, Inc.

- The demographic is the statistical data of a population, such as age, gender, education, income, and ethnicity.
- The medical office should research its strengths, weaknesses, and opportunities when developing a marketing plan. A part of this research includes assessing the competition.
- The Internet can be a strong tool for medical office advertising. Many practices manage their own Web sites, and others purchase space on a community site. There are many places to purchase advertising on the Internet.
- Many practices today have very robust Web sites, where patients are able to request or even schedule appointments, pay bills, and find answers to medical questions. These Web sites also house important patient information about the practice (i.e., biographies of physicians, insurance information).
- Direct mail advertising is any form of print advertising that is sent via the mail directly to individuals' homes. Other direct marketing initiatives include e-mail, interactive customer Web sites, promotional letters, and cell phone texting.
- Some health care facilities may choose to send direct mail advertisements directly to households, rather than through a direct mail marketing firm. Mailing lists can be purchased from marketing firms.
- In "Welcome to the Neighborhood" packets, advertisement space is often sold to businesses in the community.
- Many health care providers offer free screenings in their community as a way to bring in new patients.
- Social media sites are Internet Web sites, such as Facebook, where individuals interact on a social level; their use is becoming a popular method for medical offices to market their services.
- A focus group is a representative group of individuals brought together and questioned about their ideas on new products or services.
- Many health care providers reach out to market directly to local businesses in their community. This is a form of direct mail advertising in that advertisements may be sent to local businesses in the attempt to bring in new patients.
- Physicians sometimes offer to give educational speaking engagements in their communities. These engagements may be targeted to local businesses, or they may be targeted to local community groups.
- Advertising in the telephone directory is still done by medical practices, though it is not recommended as a primary source of advertising.
- On-hold messaging can be purchased from a vendor, or clinics can design and record their own. Because the caller is a captive audience during the hold time, this is a perfect opportunity to market items that may be of interest to the caller.
- Offering exceptional customer service to keep patients satisfied is a focus of most providers and clinics today. Patients are health care consumers, and if they are not satisfied with all aspects of their care, they may choose to seek care elsewhere.
- Patients who are very satisfied with their care will often refer their family and friends for care in the same facility. On the other hand, patients who are unhappy with their care will also discuss that fact with their family and friends, creating a negative effect on earning new business.
- Writing articles for local newspapers or periodicals is a free form of advertisement in that it costs the office nothing in money to pursue. These articles can be written on particular topics or in question-and-answer format, and they can be written by various members of the medical office staff— physicians, nurses, and medical assistants.
- Whenever a new development occurs in the medical practice, it provides a great opportunity to seek free advertisement with the local media. Examples include the addition of a new physician in the practice, a staff member who recently earned a new degree or certification, or the purchase of a new piece of equipment.
- For clinics with larger budgets for advertising, a marketing consultant or marketing firm may be hired. These companies offer all of the services listed in this chapter of your student textbook.

LEARNING ACTIVITIES

To ensure that you have achieved the learning objectives in this chapter:

1. In the Terminology Review section below, define the key terminology found in this chapter of your student text.

2. Conduct an Internet search to locate two medical offices in your local area. What features are available for patients at these two sites (e.g., appointment scheduling, online bill paying). Which, in your opinion, is the more robust of the two sites? Why?

3. Research online the types of services offered to pediatric patients on the Internet. What types of marketing materials do you believe would work best to advertise new services for this patient population?

APPLIED LEARNING EXERCISES

Using a separate sheet of paper, complete the following assignments:

1. Research the Internet and locate a physician Web design and Internet marketing firm. What are the various marketing and advertising services offered by this company?

2. Imagine you are the medical office manager of a large physician practice, and you are responsible for the marketing and advertising initiatives of the practice. How would you go about the task of advertising an upcoming free screening event? What factors would you consider in order to make the event a success?

3. Imagine that you are the office manager of an obstetrics and gynecology practice. Write a brief essay describing the types of marketing initiatives you feel would bring the medical practice the best return on investment (e.g., direct mail, television advertising).

TERMINOLOGY REVIEW

Using the glossary and highlighted terms in the textbook, define the following terms:

demographic: _____

_____

direct mail advertising: _____

_____

focus group: _____

_____

marketing budget: _____

_____

marketing firm: _____

_____

marketing plan: _____

_____

return on investment: _____

_____

screenings: _____

_____

© 2015 Pearson Education, Inc.

search engine optimization: _____

_____

social media site: _____

_____

CRITICAL THINKING QUESTIONS

1. Margaret Thompson is the office manager at the Sunnyview Medical Clinic. She is hiring the ABC Marketing Company to design and manage the clinic's Web site. What information should Margaret prepare for the marketing company so that the firm can make it available on the clinic's site?

_____

_____

_____

_____

_____

_____

2. Margaret Thompson, office manager at the Sunnyview Medical Clinic, is working with the ABC Marketing Company to offer patients special features on the clinic's Web site. What popular features might she ask the ABC Marketing Company to make available on the site?

_____

_____

_____

_____

_____

_____

3. Joseph Rodriguez, CMA (AAMA), is the office manager at the new Hyde Park Medical Group Practice. The physicians have asked him to research advertisement opportunities available through social media sites, such as Facebook. What might Joseph report back to the physicians?

_____

_____

_____

_____

_____

4. Heather Reinhart, RMA (AMT), is the office manager at the Downtown Pediatric Clinic. She is interested in gathering information from parents in the community regarding their satisfaction with the services provided. How might Heather gather this information?

_____

_____

_____

© 2015 Pearson Education, Inc.

_____

_____

_____

_____

5. Michael Benton, CMAA (NHA), is responsible for marketing and advertising in the medical clinic where he is employed. The physician has asked Michael if there is a way for the clinic to advertise its services to patients when the patients call the office. What suggestions might Michael make to the physician regarding the type of marketing available?

_____

_____

_____

_____

_____

_____

_____

CHAPTER REVIEW TEST

MULTIPLE CHOICE

Circle the letter of the correct answer.

1. Which form of advertising is sent via the mail directly to individuals' homes?
   a. Brochure
   b. Pamphlet
   c. Direct mail
   d. Billboard
   e. Television

2. _____ are Internet Web sites where individuals interact and medical offices can market their services.
   a. Search engines
   b. Service media sites
   c. Advertising sites
   d. Social media sites
   e. Marketing sites

3. A representative group of individuals brought together and questioned about their ideas on new products or services is referred to as a _____.
   a. focus group
   b. media group
   c. service group
   d. marketing group
   e. marketing firm

4. Which of the following is NOT recommended as the sole form of advertising for a medical practice?
   a. Internet
   b. Direct mail
   c. Billboard
   d. Telephone
   e. Focus group

© 2015 Pearson Education, Inc.

5. What would likely happen if a patient is unhappy with her care?
   a. She may refer her family and friends to the office.
   b. She may express her concern with a lawyer.
   c. She may choose care elsewhere.
   d. She may continue to visit the practice.
   e. None of the above.

6. All of the following questions might be included on a satisfaction survey of patients to rate their feeling on the medical practice EXCEPT:
   a. What is your ethnicity?
   b. Do you feel you were greeted in a friendly manner by the receptionist?
   c. Do you feel the medical assistant showed genuine concern for you?
   d. How do you feel about the amount of time the physician spent with you?
   e. How do you feel about the amount of time you were on hold before your call was answered?

7. A comprehensive outline of a business's overall marketing objectives in a given period is referred to as the _____.
   a. demographic
   b. advertising budget
   c. direct mail piece
   d. return on investment
   e. marketing plan

8. Which of the following is considered a costly form of advertising?
   a. Patient information pamphlets
   b. Television ad
   c. Social media advertising
   d. Focus group
   e. Informational articles

9. A Web page on which an individual records opinions and links to other sites on a regular basis is a _____.
   a. social media site
   b. search engine
   c. blog
   d. customer satisfaction site
   e. None of the above

10. Which form is typically filled out by the patient at a screening event?
    a. Customer satisfaction form
    b. HIPAA compliance form
    c. HIPAA business authorization agreement
    d. Patient history
    e. Patient registration

TRUE/FALSE

Identify whether the statement is true (T) or false (F).

_____ 1. At patient screening events, some type of patient history form is typically filled out to collect basic information about the patient and for future marketing endeavors.

_____ 2. Writing articles for local newspapers is one of the most costly forms of advertising.

_____ 3. Telephone book advertising is not recommended as the sole form of advertising for a medical practice.

_____ 4. Most small medical offices hire marketing firms to handle the office's marketing and advertising initiatives.

_____ 5. A strategic marketing group is a small group of individuals who are used to survey satisfaction with a particular service.

_____ 6. Focus groups consist of individuals from different demographics who live within the same community.

_____ 7. Many health care providers market directly to local businesses in their community.

_____ 8. In offices where there is a designated medical office manager, the physician is typically the person leading the office's marketing efforts.

_____ 9. The best preparation for beginning any marketing initiative is a properly prepared marketing plan.

_____ 10. The clinic's marketing budget is the amount of money allocated by a company to purchase equipment and supplies.

SHORT ANSWER

1. What is the role of a marketing firm in the marketing and advertising of a medical practice?

_____

_____

_____

_____

_____

2. What is a patient demographic?

_____

_____

_____

_____

_____

3. How might the medical office devise a marketing plan to target certain demographics?

_____

_____

_____

_____

_____

4. What factors should the office manager consider when researching the competition?

_____

_____

_____

_____

_____

5. How might a medical practice use the Internet for marketing purposes?

_____

_____

_____

© 2015 Pearson Education, Inc.

6. What is search engine optimization?

_____

_____

_____

_____

_____

7. How might a medical practice develop a robust Web site?

_____

_____

_____

_____

_____

8. How and why might a medical practice advertise through a "Welcome to the Neighborhood" packet?

_____

_____

_____

_____

_____

9. What should the medical office manager consider when setting up a free scoliosis screening?

_____

_____

_____

_____

_____

10. Describe how a medical office might successfully market its services by using a social media site such as Facebook.

_____

_____

_____

_____

© 2015 Pearson Education, Inc.

CHAPTER 24

The Practicum Experience and Competing in the Job Market

CHAPTER OUTLINE

Introduction

The Practicum Experience

Writing an Effective Résumé

Preparing a Cover Letter

Identifying Places to Look for Employment

Completing Employment Applications

The Successful Interview

Changing Jobs

Review

COMPETENCY SKILLS PERFORMANCE

Procedure 24-1: Write an Effective Résumé

Procedure 24-2: Compose a Cover Letter

Procedure 24-3: Follow Up after an Interview

CHAPTER REVIEW

- The practicum comes at the end of the medical assistant's training. This program offers benefits to the student, the practicum site, and the medical assisting program.

- The medical assistant should create an attractive, effective résumé and keep it updated with the most current information. The résumé must be free of typographical and grammatical errors. When résumés are clear, accurate, and written using action words, they can help medical assisting candidates secure jobs.

- When sending a résumé to a potential employer, the medical assistant should always include a cover letter. The cover letter helps the job applicant to secure an opportunity to interview for the position he or she is interested in. Cover letters support job-searching initiatives by explaining to the potential employer the reasons why the applicant is right for the job.

- Medical assistants can search for job opportunities in newspapers, at job fairs, via local medical assisting programs, and on the Internet.

© 2015 Pearson Education, Inc.

- During the interview process, the medical assistant should adhere to a professional stance and manner of dress and should always follow up after the interview with a thank-you note and/or telephone call.
- When medical assistants decide to seek new employment, they should take all steps to leave their employers on good terms. Requesting a recommendation letter upon leaving the office may help the medical assistant secure a future position.

LEARNING ACTIVITIES

To ensure that you have achieved the learning objectives in this chapter:

1. In the Terminology Review section on page 216, define the key terminology found in this chapter of your student text.

2. Create a list of action words that can be used on a résumé.

_____

_____

_____

_____

_____

_____

_____

_____

_____

_____

_____

3. Create a list of places medical assistants might look for employment in their field.

_____

_____

_____

_____

_____

4. Create a list of things you should *not* do in an interview.

_____

_____

_____

_____

_____

_____

_____

_____

_____

APPLIED LEARNING EXERCISES

Using a separate sheet of paper, complete the following assignments:

1. Speak with the faculty member in your medical assisting program who oversees the practicum program. Ask this person to describe the practicum experience, including the benefits afforded to the student, the site, and the medical assisting program. Write a 1–2 page essay describing your interview.

2. Create a résumé for yourself.

3. Create a sample cover letter.

4. Write a brief essay describing the importance of body language and proper dress during the interview.

5. Write a brief essay explaining the importance of following up after an interview, and when it should be done.

6. Write a brief essay outlining a plan of action for leaving a position on the desired terms.

TERMINOLOGY REVIEW

Using the glossary and highlighted terms in the textbook, define the following terms:

advocate: _____

_____

cover letter: _____

_____

interview: _____

_____

mentor: _____

_____

practicum: _____

_____

preceptor: _____

_____

résumé: _____

_____

CRITICAL THINKING QUESTIONS

1. William Harrison is finishing his medical assisting training and is preparing for his practicum experience. William's wife asks him what he will be doing during his practicum. How might William answer her question?

_____

_____

_____

© 2015 Pearson Education, Inc.

2. Joann Felmer is a student in an administrative medical assisting course. She has been given an assignment to describe the benefits of the practicum experience for the student medical assistant. How might Joann answer this question?

_____

_____

_____

_____

_____

3. Corey Rubatino, CMA (AAMA), has recently been hired to work for Dr. Joe Cresanti. On Corey's first day, he has been asked by Dr. Cresanti to complete a procedure he has not been trained to do. How should Corey react to this request?

_____

_____

_____

_____

_____

4. Maggie Levinski, RMA (AMT), is the program director in an accredited medical assisting program. She is attempting to add additional practicum sites to the program roster. When Maggie meets with a potential site, she is asked to explain the benefits of the program to the practicum site. How might Maggie answer this question?

_____

_____

_____

_____

5. Jason Ripper is a student medical assistant going out to his practicum site for the first time. When he arrives at the site, the office manager asks Jason to sign a HIPAA agreement before Jason can begin work. Jason asks the office manager to explain why this form is needed. How might the office manager answer?

_____

_____

_____

_____

CHAPTER REVIEW TEST

MULTIPLE CHOICE

Circle the letter of the correct answer.

1. The _____ is the individual who will serve as an on-site resource to the student medical assistant during the practicum.

   a. mentor
   b. office manager
   c. physician
   d. practicum coordinator
   e. None of the above

2. Which of the following is NOT a responsibility of the student medical assistant during the practicum?

   a. Be on time
   b. Dress appropriately
   c. Act in a professional manner
   d. Diagnose patients
   e. Be prepared

3. The _____ is primarily responsible for choosing appropriate practicum sites for students.

   a. physician
   b. advocate
   c. office manager
   d. practicum coordinator
   e. medical assisting student

4. When a student medical assistant has a concern about something at the practicum site, to whose attention should the student bring the problem?

   a. A coworker
   b. The student's spouse
   c. The practicum coordinator
   d. The dean of the college
   e. The patient

5. Which of the following is a reason why the medical assistant may not be called for an interview?

   a. The résumé contains typographical errors.
   b. The résumé contains grammatical errors.
   c. The résumé contains crossed-out words and handwritten corrections.
   d. The résumé is printed on lime-green paper.
   e. All of the above

6. A résumé should ideally be _____ pages in length.

   a. 1–2
   b. 2–3
   c. 3–4
   d. 4–5
   e. There is no page limit requirement for a résumé.

7. The medical assistant may inquire about salary _____.

   a. in the résumé
   b. in the cover letter
   c. in the followup letter
   d. at the first interview
   e. once the position has been offered

© 2015 Pearson Education, Inc.

8. All of the following is true of the practicum experience EXCEPT _____.

   a. the medical assisting student will receive a salary and benefits

   b. every accredited medical assisting program ends with a practicum program

   c. some students are offered employment at the end of their practicum

   d. the medical assisting student is not paid for the practicum work but will earn credit toward graduation from the medical assisting program

   e. the practicum experience benefits the student as well as the medical assisting program

9. All of the following are considered acceptable during the interview EXCEPT _____.

   a. requesting parking validation

   b. arriving a bit early

   c. taking notes

   d. asking questions

   e. None of the above are acceptable during the interview.

10. When it comes time to interview, the candidate should bring _____ copy (copies) of the résumé to the interview.

   a. one

   b. two

   c. three

   d. four

   e. It is not necessary to bring extra copies of the résumé to the interview.

TRUE/FALSE

Identify whether the statement is true (T) or false (F).

_____ 1. Many medical assisting practicum coordinators visit the student medical assistants while at their practicum site.

_____ 2. Many medical assistants are asked to log their learning experiences while at the practicum site.

_____ 3. The résumé should list the reasons why the applicant left his or her former job(s).

_____ 4. The résumé should list any reasons why the applicant may not be able to perform the job, such as lack of transportation or unreliable child care.

_____ 5. If the applicant can speak languages other than English fluently, that skill should be listed on the résumé.

_____ 6. Résumés should contain the e-mail address of the applicant.

_____ 7. The information on the résumé should be exaggerated in order to make the applicant seem as skilled as possible.

_____ 8. The cover letter is a link between the résumé and the open job.

_____ 9. Many employers will ask potential employees to fill out employment applications, even if the employee has already submitted a résumé.

_____ 10. If a section on an employment application does not apply, the applicant should leave the section blank.

SHORT ANSWER

1. What items should be included on a résumé?

_____

_____

_____

_____

_____

2. What is the role of the practicum coordinator in the practicum experience?

_____

_____

_____

_____

3. What is the purpose of a cover letter?

_____

_____

_____

_____

4. Why should an applicant research the office he or she will be interviewing with prior to the interview?

_____

_____

_____

_____

5. Why is it predicted that the medical assisting profession will grow over the next ten years?

_____

_____

_____

_____

6. Describe the appropriate attire that should be worn for an interview.

_____

_____

_____

_____

7. Describe the purpose of following up after an interview. Include the ways an applicant might follow up after an interview.

_____

_____

_____

_____

© 2015 Pearson Education, Inc.

8. When is it appropriate for the medical assistant to discuss salary with a prospective employer?

_____

_____

_____

_____

9. When changes are needed on the résumé, how should the applicant make those changes?

_____

_____

_____

_____

10. If an employer asks an illegal question during the interview, how should the applicant respond?

_____

_____

_____

_____

Competency Check-Offs

AFFECTIVE BEHAVIORS

Affective behaviors are very important to the role of medical assisting. These behaviors display sensitivity to the patient, convey an understanding of laws and regulations, and also provide an overall professional component to the medical assisting profession.

The weighed competencies in the student workbook vary slightly from the competencies presented in the textbook. The competencies within this appendix place an emphasis on affective behaviors by showing them in a ***bold and italicized*** font. Note that not all procedures will have affective behaviors.

Your instructors will expect to see these behaviors demonstrated during the performance of a procedure, as necessary. Failure to exhibit these affective behaviors will result in a loss of points associated with the point value of the given step. It is essential to review the weighted competencies found in the workbook prior to being tested and graded.

© 2015 Pearson Education, Inc.

Name: _____

Date: _____

Procedure 2-1:

Adapt to Change

Objective: To adapt to change when given a new task within the time limit set by the instructor.

Supplies: Notepad and pen.

Affective Behaviors: Affective behaviors provide a professional approach to a skill that enhances the patient encounter. These behaviors may also display sensitivity to patients' rights, enhance communication, convey an understanding of laws and regulations, and/or provide an overall professional component to the medical assisting profession. Pay close attention to these skills, which appear in ***bold, italicized*** font.

Notes to the Student:

_____

_____

_____

_____

_____

_____

Skills Assessment Requirements

Read and familiarize yourself with the procedure; complete the minimum practice requirements (MPRs). Document each MPR using proper charting technique. Complete each procedure within a reasonable amount of time, with a minimum of 85 percent accuracy.

© 2015 Pearson Education, Inc.

Name: _____

Date: _____

POINT VALUE ◆ = 3–6 points ★ = 7–9 points		PRACTICE TRIAL	GRADED TRIAL #1	GRADED TRIAL #2	NOTES:
1. ◆	*Listen closely* as a new task is requested.				
2. ◆	Ask questions to clarify the request, if needed.				
3. ◆	Take notes about the task, if needed.				
4. ★	Begin working on the new task while *maintaining a positive and professional attitude*.				

© 2015 Pearson Education, Inc.

Name: _____

Date: _____

Document: Enter the appropriate information in the chart below.

Grading

Points Earned	_____		
Points Possible	_____	27	27
Percent Grade (Points Earned/Points Possible)	_____		
PASS:	_____	❏ YES ❏ NO ❏ N/A	❏ YES ❏ NO ❏ N/A

Instructor Sign-Off

Instructor: _____ Date: _____

© 2015 Pearson Education, Inc.

Procedure 4-1:

Prepare an Informed Consent for Treatment Form

Objective: Prepare an informed consent for treatment form correctly within the time limit set by the instructor.

Supplies: Informed consent for treatment form, blue or black ink pen, copy machine.

Affective Behaviors: Affective behaviors provide a professional approach to a skill that enhances the patient encounter. These behaviors may also display sensitivity to patients' rights, enhance communication, convey an understanding of laws and regulations, and/or provide an overall professional component to the medical assisting profession. Pay close attention to these skills, which appear in **bold, italicized** font.

Notes to the Student:

_____

_____

_____

_____

_____

_____

Skills Assessment Requirements

Read and familiarize yourself with the procedure; complete the minimum practice requirements (MPRs). Document each MPR using proper charting technique. Complete each procedure within a reasonable amount of time, with a minimum of 85 percent accuracy.

© 2015 Pearson Education, Inc.

POINT VALUE ◆ = 3–6 points ★ = 7–9 points		PRACTICE TRIAL	GRADED TRIAL #1	GRADED TRIAL #2	NOTES:
1. ★	As the physician goes over the details of the upcoming procedure with the patient, fill in the informed consent form. The form must include: • The name of the procedure or treatment to be performed. • The expected benefits of the procedure. • Any possible risks of the procedure. • Any accepted alternatives to the procedure and the risks or benefits associated with each. • The fact that the patient may choose to forgo the procedure and the possible risks or benefits associated with that choice. **Double check this information for accuracy.**				
2. ◆	Be certain the form lists the patient's name, birthdate, and the place the procedure is to be performed (in office, hospital, etc.). **Double check this information for accuracy.**				
3. ◆	Show the consent form to the physician for him or her to verify all information is correct.				

© 2015 Pearson Education, Inc.

Name: _____

Date: _____

4. ★	After the physician has left the room, go over the form with the patient. If the patient has further questions about the procedure, have the patient wait in the treatment room while you ask the physician to return to answer the questions. If the patient has no further questions about the procedure, have the patient sign the consent form.				
5. ◆	Sign the consent form as a witness to the patient's signature.				
6. ◆	Go over any specifics with the patient about the procedure day, such as any restrictions to eating or drinking on the day of the surgery, or where the patient should park his or her car.				
7. ◆	Make a copy of the consent form for the patient. Place the original form in the patient's file.				

© 2015 Pearson Education, Inc.

Document: Enter the appropriate information in the chart below.

Grading

Points Earned	_____		
Points Possible	_____	48	48
Percent Grade (Points Earned/Points Possible)	_____		
PASS:	_____	❏ YES ❏ NO ❏ N/A	❏ YES ❏ NO ❏ N/A

Instructor Sign-Off

Instructor: _____   **Date:** _____

© 2015 Pearson Education, Inc.

Procedure 4-2:

Obtain Authorization for the Release of Patient Medical Records

Objective: Correctly obtain an authorization from a patient to release information within the time limit set by the instructor.

Supplies: Release-of-records authorization form, blue or black ink pen, copy machine, patient medical record.

Affective Behaviors: Affective behaviors provide a professional approach to a skill that enhances the patient encounter. These behaviors may also display sensitivity to patients' rights, enhance communication, convey an understanding of laws and regulations, and/or provide an overall professional component to the medical assisting profession. Pay close attention to these skills, which appear in **bold, italicized** font.

Notes to the Student:

_____

_____

_____

_____

_____

_____

Skills Assessment Requirements

Read and familiarize yourself with the procedure; complete the minimum practice requirements (MPRs). Document each MPR using proper charting technique. Complete each procedure within a reasonable amount of time, with a minimum of 85 percent accuracy.

© 2015 Pearson Education, Inc.

Name: _____

Date: _____

POINT VALUE ◆ = 3–6 points ★ = 7–9 points		PRACTICE TRIAL	GRADED TRIAL #1	GRADED TRIAL #2	NOTES:
1. ★	When the patient states all or a portion of the patient's record is to be released to a third party, ask the patient to sign and date a release-of-records form.				
2. ◆	Verify the address where the patient would like the copies of the record sent.				
3. ◆	Verify the records the patient would like released. If the patient requests specific release dates, ask the patient to write those dates on the release-of-records form.				
4. ◆	Verify if the patient would like super-protected information to be released (HIV/AIDS, mental health, drug or alcohol rehabilitation information, sexually transmitted disease information, or information about family planning), and ask the patient to check the appropriate box on the authorization form to allow the release of that information.				
5. ★	Identify which information in the medical record must be copied.				
6. ◆	Copy the appropriate documents from the medical record. **To protect patient privacy, verify all of the patient's medical record has been removed from the copy machine.**				
7. ◆	Send the copies to the requested location.				
8. ◆	Make a notation of the release of information in the patient's medical record.				

© 2015 Pearson Education, Inc.

Name: _____

Date: _____

Document: Enter the appropriate information in the chart below.

Grading

Points Earned	_____		
Points Possible	_____	54	54
Percent Grade (Points Earned/Points Possible)	_____		
PASS:	_____	❏ YES ❏ NO ❏ N/A	❏ YES ❏ NO ❏ N/A

Instructor Sign-Off

Instructor: _____ **Date:** _____

© 2015 Pearson Education, Inc.

Name: _____

Date: _____

Procedure 4-3:

Respond to a Request for Copies of a Patient's Medical Record

Objective: Respond to a request for copies of a patient's medical record correctly within the time limit set by the instructor.

Supplies: Release-of-records authorization form, blue or black ink pen, copy machine, patient's medical record.

Affective Behaviors: Affective behaviors provide a professional approach to a skill that enhances the patient encounter. These behaviors may also display sensitivity to patients' rights, enhance communication, convey an understanding of laws and regulations, and/or provide an overall professional component to the medical assisting profession. Pay close attention to these skills, which appear in **bold, italicized** font.

Notes to the Student:

_____

_____

_____

_____

_____

_____

Skills Assessment Requirements

Read and familiarize yourself with the procedure; complete the minimum practice requirements (MPRs). Document each MPR using proper charting technique. Complete each procedure within a reasonable amount of time, with a minimum of 85 percent accuracy.

© 2015 Pearson Education, Inc.

Name: _____

Date: _____

POINT VALUE ◆ = 3–6 points ★ = 7–9 points	PRACTICE TRIAL	GRADED TRIAL #1	GRADED TRIAL #2	NOTES:
1. ★ Verify that the release-of-records form has been signed and dated by the patient or the patient's legal representative.				
2. ◆ **Carefully review the release form for any specific date or information requests.**				
3. ◆ Check if the patient has authorized release of super-protected information (HIV/AIDS, mental health, drug or alcohol rehabilitation information, sexually transmitted disease information, or information about family planning).				
4. ◆ Verify that you have pulled the correct patient file.				
5. ◆ Locate the documents to be copied.				
6. ★ Review the documents to be copied to verify that they carry the correct patient name and contain the information requested in the authorization to release information and only that information.				
7. ◆ Copy the appropriate documents.				
8. ◆ Send the copies to the requesting agency.				
9. ★ File the release-of-records request in the patient's medical record with a notation of the documents that were copied and sent.				

© 2015 Pearson Education, Inc.

Name: _____

Date: _____

Document: Enter the appropriate information in the chart below.

Grading

Points Earned	_____		
Points Possible	_____	63	63
Percent Grade (Points Earned/Points Possible)	_____		
PASS:	_____	❏ YES ❏ NO ❏ N/A	❏ YES ❏ NO ❏ N/A

Instructor Sign-Off

Instructor: _____   **Date:** _____

© 2015 Pearson Education, Inc.

Name: _____

Date: _____

Procedure 6-1:

Use Effective Listening Skills in Patient Interviews

Objective: To use effective listening skills in interviewing the patient correctly within the time limit set by the instructor.

Supplies: Patient history form and pen.

Affective Behaviors: Affective behaviors provide a professional approach to a skill that enhances the patient encounter. These behaviors may also display sensitivity to patients' rights, enhance communication, convey an understanding of laws and regulations, and/or provide an overall professional component to the medical assisting profession. Pay close attention to these skills, which appear in **bold, *italicized*** font.

Notes to the Student:

_____

_____

_____

_____

_____

_____

Skills Assessment Requirements

Read and familiarize yourself with the procedure; complete the minimum practice requirements (MPRs). Document each MPR using proper charting technique. Complete each procedure within a reasonable amount of time, with a minimum of 85 percent accuracy.

Name: _____

Date: _____

POINT VALUE ◆ = 3–6 points ★ = 7–9 points		PRACTICE TRIAL	GRADED TRIAL #1	GRADED TRIAL #2	NOTES:
1. ◆	*Smile, and introduce yourself to the patient.*				
2. ★	Identify the patient by verifying the patient's birth date.				
3. ★	Verify that you have the correct patient chart.				
4. ◆	Maintain a professional persona.				
5. ◆	*Maintain eye contact with the patient.*				
6. ◆	Ask the patient open-ended questions.				
7. ◆	Do not interrupt the patient.				
8. ◆	Paraphrase the patient's statements to verify comprehension.				
9. ◆	*Watch for the patient's nonverbal communication.*				
10. ◆	*Summarize the patient's statements and conclude the interview.*				
11. ★	Document appropriate information in the patient's file.				

© 2015 Pearson Education, Inc.

Name: _____

Date: _____

Document: Enter the appropriate information in the chart below.

Grading

Points Earned	_____		
Points Possible	_____	75	75
Percent Grade (Points Earned/Points Possible)	_____		
PASS:	_____	❑ YES ❑ NO ❑ N/A	❑ YES ❑ NO ❑ N/A

Instructor Sign-Off

Instructor: _____ **Date:** _____

Procedure 6-2:

Communicate with a Hearing-Impaired Patient

Objective: Communicate with a hearing-impaired patient correctly within the time limit set by the instructor.

Supplies: Patient's paper or electronic medical record and blue or black ink pen.

Affective Behaviors: Affective behaviors provide a professional approach to a skill that enhances the patient encounter. These behaviors may also display sensitivity to patients' rights, enhance communication, convey an understanding of laws and regulations, and/or provide an overall professional component to the medical assisting profession. Pay close attention to these skills, which appear in **_bold, italicized_** font.

Notes to the Student:

_____

_____

_____

_____

_____

_____

Skills Assessment Requirements

Read and familiarize yourself with the procedure; complete the minimum practice requirements (MPRs). Document each MPR using proper charting technique. Complete each procedure within a reasonable amount of time, with a minimum of 85 percent accuracy.

© 2015 Pearson Education, Inc.

Name: _____

Date: _____

POINT VALUE ◆ = 3–6 points ★ = 7–9 points		PRACTICE TRIAL	GRADED TRIAL #1	GRADED TRIAL #2	NOTES:
1. ◆	Alert the patient that you are ready to take him to the examination room by entering the reception area, touching the patient's arm to get his attention, and motioning him to follow.				
2. ◆	If the patient has an interpreter, also have the interpreter enter the examination room.				
3. ★	**When speaking, look directly at the patient and speak slowly.**				
4. ◆	When the patient can read lips, verify understanding through patient questioning. **When comprehension is lacking, write instructions for the patient.**				
5. ◆	When asking a patient to change into a gown, ask the patient to flip a switch or crack the door open when ready. People with hearing impairments cannot hear a knock to announce the physician's arrival.				
6. ★	At the end of the patient's visit, chart all communications, including verification of the patient's understanding.				

© 2015 Pearson Education, Inc.

Name: _____

Date: _____

Document: Enter the appropriate information in the chart below.

Grading

Points Earned	_____		
Points Possible	_____	42	42
Percent Grade (Points Earned/Points Possible)	_____		
PASS:	_____	❏ YES ❏ NO ❏ N/A	❏ YES ❏ NO ❏ N/A

Instructor Sign-Off

Instructor: _____ **Date:** _____

© 2015 Pearson Education, Inc.

Procedure 6-3:

Communicate with a Sight-Impaired Patient

Objective: Communicate with a sight-impaired patient correctly within the time limit set by the instructor.

Supplies: Patient's paper or electronic file and blue or black ink pen.

Affective Behaviors: Affective behaviors provide a professional approach to a skill that enhances the patient encounter. These behaviors may also display sensitivity to patients' rights, enhance communication, convey an understanding of laws and regulations, and/or provide an overall professional component to the medical assisting profession. Pay close attention to these skills, which appear in **bold, *italicized*** font.

Notes to the Student:

_____

_____

_____

_____

_____

_____

Skills Assessment Requirements

Read and familiarize yourself with the procedure; complete the minimum practice requirements (MPRs). Document each MPR using proper charting technique. Complete each procedure within a reasonable amount of time, with a minimum of 85 percent accuracy.

© 2015 Pearson Education, Inc.

Name: _____

Date: _____

POINT VALUE ◆ = 3–6 points ★ = 7–9 points		PRACTICE TRIAL	GRADED TRIAL #1	GRADED TRIAL #2	NOTES:
1. ◆	*Alert the patient that you are ready to visit the examination room by entering the reception area, touching the patient's arm, and offering your arm for the patient to hold.*				
2. ◆	Ensure that the patient's service animal accompanies him to the examination room.				
3. ★	Alert the patient to any steps, doorways, ramps, or slopes along the way.				
4. ◆	Take the patient to a private area, outside of other patients' views or hearing ranges.				
5. ◆	Place the patient's hand on the chair or table where you would like him to sit. *Ensure that the patient is comfortable by asking, "Do you feel comfortable?"*				
6. ◆	Arrange for any service animal to sit directly next to the patient.				
7. ◆	Ask the patient the questions on the history form, and write down the answers. *Ensure the patient's responses are clearly understood and verify information obtained.*				

© 2015 Pearson Education, Inc.

8. ★	At the end of the patient's visit, chart all communications, including how the patient's understanding was verified.				
9. ★	Sign and date the patient history form, and note that the history form was completed for the patient due to sight impairment.				

© 2015 Pearson Education, Inc.

Name: _____

Date: _____

Document: Enter the appropriate information in the chart below.

Grading

Points Earned	_____		
Points Possible	_____	63	63
Percent Grade (Points Earned/Points Possible)	_____		
PASS:	_____	❏ YES ❏ NO ❏ N/A	❏ YES ❏ NO ❏ N/A

Instructor Sign-Off

Instructor: _____   **Date:** _____

© 2015 Pearson Education, Inc.

Name: _____

Date: _____

Procedure 6-4:

Communicate with a Patient via Interpreter

Objective: Communicate with a patient via an interpreter correctly within the time limit set by the instructor.

Supplies: Patient's paper or electronic file and blue or black ink pen.

Affective Behaviors: Affective behaviors provide a professional approach to a skill that enhances the patient encounter. These behaviors may also display sensitivity to patients' rights, enhance communication, convey an understanding of laws and regulations, and/or provide an overall professional component to the medical assisting profession. Pay close attention to these skills, which appear in **bold, italicized** font.

Notes to the Student:

_____

_____

_____

_____

_____

_____

_____

Skills Assessment Requirements

Read and familiarize yourself with the procedure; complete the minimum practice requirements (MPRs). Document each MPR using proper charting technique. Complete each procedure within a reasonable amount of time, with a minimum of 85 percent accuracy.

© 2015 Pearson Education, Inc.

Name: _____

Date: _____

POINT VALUE ◆ = 3–6 points ★ = 7–9 points		PRACTICE TRIAL	GRADED TRIAL #1	GRADED TRIAL #2	NOTES:
1. ◆	When the patient arrives in the office with an interpreter, obtain the name of the interpreter and verify the spelling.				
2. ★	**Obtain the interpreter's contact information for the patient's medical record.** If the interpreter has a business card, attach it to the patient's file.				
3. ◆	Communicate with the patient directly; **do not speak directly to the interpreter.**				
4. ◆	When any of the interpreter's comments are unclear, **ask for clarification. Ask the patient if she has any questions prior to leaving the room.**				
5. ★	Document all essential parts of the interview in the patient's chart.				

© 2015 Pearson Education, Inc.

Name: _____

Date: _____

Document: Enter the appropriate information in the chart below.

Grading

Points Earned	_____		
Points Possible	_____	36	36
Percent Grade (Points Earned/Points Possible)	_____		
PASS:	_____	❏ YES ❏ NO ❏ N/A	❏ YES ❏ NO ❏ N/A

Instructor Sign-Off

Instructor: _____ **Date:** _____

© 2015 Pearson Education, Inc.

Name: _____

Date: _____

Procedure 6-5:

Prepare a Patient's Specialist Referral

Objective: Prepare a referral for a patient to see a specialist correctly within the time limit set by the instructor.

Supplies: Telephone, blue or black ink pen or electronic medical record, patient's paper or electronic file, referral form to a specialist.

Affective Behaviors: Affective behaviors provide a professional approach to a skill that enhances the patient encounter. These behaviors may also display sensitivity to patients' rights, enhance communication, convey an understanding of laws and regulations, and/or provide an overall professional component to the medical assisting profession. Pay close attention to these skills, which appear in **bold, *italicized*** font.

Notes to the Student:

_____

_____

_____

_____

_____

_____

Skills Assessment Requirements

Read and familiarize yourself with the procedure; complete the minimum practice requirements (MPRs). Document each MPR using proper charting technique. Complete each procedure within a reasonable amount of time, with a minimum of 85 percent accuracy.

Name: _____

Date: _____

POINT VALUE ◆ = 3–6 points ★ = 7–9 points		PRACTICE TRIAL	GRADED TRIAL #1	GRADED TRIAL #2	NOTES:
1. ★	Verify the patient file is correct.				
2. ◆	Verify the referral form for the specialist is correct.				
3. ◆	Verify the doctor's instructions (e.g., What does the doctor want the patient to be seen for? How soon does the patient need to be seen?).				
4. ◆	**Choose a private location, out of the hearing range of other patients.**				
5. ◆	If the pending referral is not an emergency and the patient is in the clinic, ask the patient for a convenient time of day to see the specialist.				
6. ◆	Call the specialist's office, and ask to speak to the person who handles the schedule.				
7. ◆	**Warmly greet and identify yourself to the person on the other end of the phone.** Provide personal identification and the name of the referring doctor or clinic.				
8. ◆	State the reason for the call.				
9. ◆	Give patient information as requested by the specialist's office. **Only provide the information necessary for the purpose of the referral.**				
10. ◆	Set an appointment date and time. If the patient is in the clinic, verify the date and time.				
11. ◆	Document the appointment's date and time on the referral form. If the patient is in the clinic, give the patient the referral form. Choose to mail the referral form when there is time before the appointment.				
12. ★	Document the call's results in the patient's chart.				

© 2015 Pearson Education, Inc.

Name: _____

Date: _____

Document: Enter the appropriate information in the chart below.

Grading

Points Earned	_____		
Points Possible	_____	78	78
Percent Grade (Points Earned/Points Possible)	_____		
PASS:	_____	❏ YES ❏ NO ❏ N/A	❏ YES ❏ NO ❏ N/A

Instructor Sign-Off

Instructor: _____ **Date:** _____

© 2015 Pearson Education, Inc.

Procedure 6-6:

Identify Community Resources

Objective: To identify community resources correctly within the time limit set by the instructor.

Supplies: A computer with Internet access, written pamphlets and brochures, telephone directories.

Notes to the Student:

_____

_____

_____

_____

_____

_____

Skills Assessment Requirements

Read and familiarize yourself with the procedure; complete the minimum practice requirements (MPRs). Document each MPR using proper charting technique. Complete each procedure within a reasonable amount of time, with a minimum of 85 percent accuracy.

© 2015 Pearson Education, Inc.

Name: _____

Date: _____

POINT VALUE ◆ = 3–6 points ★ = 7–9 points		PRACTICE TRIAL	GRADED TRIAL #1	GRADED TRIAL #2	NOTES:
1. ★	Locate the name, address, telephone number, and Web site address for each of the following need categories in your community: • Homeless services • HIV/AIDS resources • Disability services • Domestic violence services • Public assistance • Housing authority/services • Ombudsman services • Foster care for children • Foster care for adults • Senior services • Legal aid • Rape victim services • Crime victim services • Culturally specific services (Native American, military, etc.) • Medical assistant services (Medicaid, etc.)				
2. ◆	Identify at least one to three resources for each category.				
3. ★	Create a written document to give to patients.				

© 2015 Pearson Education, Inc.

Name: _____

Date: _____

Document: Enter the appropriate information in the chart below.

Grading

Points Earned	_____		
Points Possible	_____	24	24
Percent Grade (Points Earned/Points Possible)	_____		
PASS:	_____	❏ YES ❏ NO ❏ N/A	❏ YES ❏ NO ❏ N/A

Instructor Sign-Off

Instructor: _____ Date: _____

© 2015 Pearson Education, Inc.

Procedure 6-7:

Use the Internet to Find Patient Education Materials

Objective: Use the Internet to find patient education materials correctly within the time limit set by the instructor.

Supplies: Computer and printer, paper or electronic patient chart, blue or black ink pen or electronic medical record.

Affective Behaviors: Affective behaviors provide a professional approach to a skill that enhances the patient encounter. These behaviors may also display sensitivity to patients' rights, enhance communication, convey an understanding of laws and regulations, and/or provide an overall professional component to the medical assisting profession. Pay close attention to these skills, which appear in **_bold, italicized_** font.

Notes to the Student: _____

_____

_____

_____

_____

_____

_____

Skills Assessment Requirements

Read and familiarize yourself with the procedure; complete the minimum practice requirements (MPRs). Document each MPR using proper charting technique. Complete each procedure within a reasonable amount of time, with a minimum of 85 percent accuracy.

© 2015 Pearson Education, Inc.

POINT VALUE ◆ = 3–6 points ★ = 7–9 points		PRACTICE TRIAL	GRADED TRIAL #1	GRADED TRIAL #2	NOTES:
1. ◆	Using the computer, *locate reputable Web sites for desired materials.*				
2. ◆	Print copies of materials.				
3. ★	Show materials to the physician for approval.				
4. ◆	Give/mail the materials to the patient.				
5. ◆	Explain the materials to the patient as needed.				
6. ◆	Place a copy or scan the materials into the patient's file.				
7. ★	Document how the materials were given to the patient and any verbal education provided with the materials.				

© 2015 Pearson Education, Inc.

Name: _____

Date: _____

Document: Enter the appropriate information in the chart below.

Grading

Points Earned	_____		
Points Possible	_____	48	48
Percent Grade (Points Earned/Points Possible)	_____		
PASS:	_____	❑ YES ❑ NO ❑ N/A	❑ YES ❑ NO ❑ N/A

Instructor Sign-Off

Instructor: _____ **Date:** _____

© 2015 Pearson Education, Inc.

Procedure 7-1:

Compose a Business Letter

Objective: Compose a business letter correctly within the time limit set by the instructor.

Supplies: Computer with word-processing software, information for the letter.

Affective Behaviors: Affective behaviors provide a professional approach to a skill that enhances the patient encounter. These behaviors may also display sensitivity to patients' rights, enhance communication, convey an understanding of laws and regulations, and/or provide an overall professional component to the medical assisting profession. Pay close attention to these skills, which appear in **_bold, italicized_** font.

Notes to the Student:

_____

_____

_____

_____

_____

_____

Skills Assessment Requirements

Read and familiarize yourself with the procedure; complete the minimum practice requirements (MPRs). Document each MPR using proper charting technique. Complete each procedure within a reasonable amount of time, with a minimum of 85 percent accuracy.

© 2015 Pearson Education, Inc.

Name: _____

Date: _____

POINT VALUE ◆ = 3–6 points ★ = 7–9 points		PRACTICE TRIAL	GRADED TRIAL #1	GRADED TRIAL #2	NOTES:
1. ◆	Determine the recipient and content of the letter.				
2. ◆	Using the word-processing software, type the date of the letter.				
3. ◆	Type the recipient of the letter.				
4. ◆	Type the subject line.				
5. ◆	Type the greeting of the letter.				
6. ◆	Type the body of the letter. **Consider the recipient's level of understanding when communicating.**				
7. ◆	Type the salutation.				
8. ◆	Indicate enclosures, if any.				
9. ◆	Indicate if a copy of the letter will be sent to another party.				
10. ◆	Enter the initials of the letter's author, followed by your initials as the typist.				
11. ★	Perform complete electronic spelling and grammar checks.				
12. ◆	Print the letter.				
13. ★	**On paper, perform manual spelling and grammar checks.**				
14. ★	Give the letter to the physician for a signature.				
15. ◆	Address an envelope.				
16. ◆	Send the letter.				

© 2015 Pearson Education, Inc.

Name: _____

Date: _____

Document: Enter the appropriate information in the chart below.

Grading

Points Earned	_____		
Points Possible	_____	105	105
Percent Grade (Points Earned/Points Possible)	_____		
PASS:	_____	❑ YES ❑ NO ❑ N/A	❑ YES ❑ NO ❑ N/A

Instructor Sign-Off

Instructor: _____ **Date:** _____

© 2015 Pearson Education, Inc.

Name: _____

Date: _____

Procedure 7-2:

Send a Letter to a Patient about a Missed Appointment

Objective: Correctly send a letter to a patient regarding a missed appointment within the time limit set by the instructor.

Supplies: Computer with word-processing software, patient medical record.

Affective Behaviors: Affective behaviors provide a professional approach to a skill that enhances the patient encounter. These behaviors may also display sensitivity to patients' rights, enhance communication, convey an understanding of laws and regulations, and/or provide an overall professional component to the medical assisting profession. Pay close attention to these skills, which appear in **bold, italicized** font.

Notes to the Student:

_____

_____

_____

_____

_____

_____

Skills Assessment Requirements

Read and familiarize yourself with the procedure; complete the minimum practice requirements (MPRs). Document each MPR using proper charting technique. Complete each procedure within a reasonable amount of time, with a minimum of 85 percent accuracy.

© 2015 Pearson Education, Inc.

POINT VALUE ◆ = 3–6 points ★ = 7–9 points		PRACTICE TRIAL	GRADED TRIAL #1	GRADED TRIAL #2	NOTES:
1. ◆	Using the word-processing software, type the date at the top of the letter.				
2. ◆	Type the patient's name and mailing address.				
3. ◆	Type the salutation.				
4. ◆	For the subject line, type "RE: Missed Appointment."				
5. ◆	In the body of the letter, describe the appointment that was missed, including its date. **Maintain politeness in the tone of the letter.**				
6. ★	Per the physician's instructions or office policy, list the reasons the patient should call to reschedule the missed appointment.				
7. ★	Type the closing and the physician's name.				
8. ◆	Obtain the signature of the letter's author (yours or the physician's).				
9. ◆	Copy the letter for the patient's file.				
10. ◆	Send the patient the original letter.				

© 2015 Pearson Education, Inc.

Name: _____

Date: _____

Document: Enter the appropriate information in the chart below.

Grading

Points Earned	_____		
Points Possible	_____	66	66
Percent Grade (Points Earned/Points Possible)	_____		
PASS:	_____	❑ YES ❑ NO ❑ N/A	❑ YES ❑ NO ❑ N/A

Instructor Sign-Off

Instructor: _____ Date: _____

© 2015 Pearson Education, Inc.

Procedure 7-3:

Proofread Written Documents

Objective: Proofread a written document correctly within the time limit set by the instructor.

Supplies: Computer document to be proofread, computer with word-processing software.

Notes to the Student:

_____

_____

_____

_____

_____

_____

_____

Skills Assessment Requirements

Read and familiarize yourself with the procedure; complete the minimum practice requirements (MPRs). Document each MPR using proper charting technique. Complete each procedure within a reasonable amount of time, with a minimum of 85 percent accuracy.

© 2015 Pearson Education, Inc.

Name: _____

Date: _____

POINT VALUE ♦ = 3–6 points ★ = 7–9 points		PRACTICE TRIAL	GRADED TRIAL #1	GRADED TRIAL #2	NOTES:
1. ♦	Open the document using the word-processing software.				
2. ♦	Use the word processor's spelling and grammar checking functions.				
3. ♦	Save any changes.				
4. ★	Starting at the top, read the entire document to verify that all spelling, punctuation, and grammatical errors were corrected.				
5. ♦	Save any changes.				
6. ♦	Print the document.				
7. ★	Review the entire document to verify that all spelling, punctuation, and grammatical errors were corrected. If changes are made, reprint the document.				
8. ♦	Give the document to the physician for signature.				

© 2015 Pearson Education, Inc.

Name: _____

Date: _____

Document: Enter the appropriate information in the chart below.

Grading

Points Earned	_____		
Points Possible	_____	54	54
Percent Grade (Points Earned/Points Possible)	_____		
PASS:	_____	❑ YES ❑ NO ❑ N/A	❑ YES ❑ NO ❑ N/A

Instructor Sign-Off

Instructor: _____ **Date:** _____

© 2015 Pearson Education, Inc.

Procedure 7-4:

Prepare a Document for Photocopying

Objective: Prepare a document for photocopying correctly within the time limit set by the instructor.

Supplies: Photocopier, document to be copied, envelope, patient medical record.

Affective Behaviors: Affective behaviors provide a professional approach to a skill that enhances the patient encounter. These behaviors may also display sensitivity to patients' rights, enhance communication, convey an understanding of laws and regulations, and/or provide an overall professional component to the medical assisting profession. Pay close attention to these skills, which appear in **bold, italicized** font.

Notes to the Student:

_____

_____

_____

_____

_____

_____

_____

Skills Assessment Requirements

Read and familiarize yourself with the procedure; complete the minimum practice requirements (MPRs). Document each MPR using proper charting technique. Complete each procedure within a reasonable amount of time, with a minimum of 85 percent accuracy.

© 2015 Pearson Education, Inc.

Name: _____

Date: _____

POINT VALUE ◆ = 3–6 points ★ = 7–9 points		PRACTICE TRIAL	GRADED TRIAL #1	GRADED TRIAL #2	NOTES:
1. ◆	Turn the photocopy machine on and allow time for it to warm up.				
2. ◆	Place the document to be copied face down on the glass surface of the photo-copier, following the diagram on the photocopier.				
3. ◆	Indicate the number of cop-ies needed by entering the number in the appropriate place on the photocopier. ***If too many copies are accidently made, shred the extra documents.***				
4. ◆	Press the "copy" button on the photocopier.				
5. ★	Once the copy has been made, remove the original.				
6. ◆	Place the original docu-ment into an envelope to be mailed to the patient.				
7. ★	Place the photocopy of the document into the patient's file.				

© 2015 Pearson Education, Inc.

Name: _____

Date: _____

Document: Enter the appropriate information in the chart below.

Grading

Points Earned	_____		
Points Possible	_____	48	48
Percent Grade (Points Earned/Points Possible)	_____		
PASS:	_____	❏ YES ❏ NO ❏ N/A	❏ YES ❏ NO ❏ N/A

Instructor Sign-Off

Instructor: _____ **Date:** _____

© 2015 Pearson Education, Inc.

Procedure 7-5:

Fold Documents for Window Envelopes

Objective: Fold a document for use with a window envelope correctly within the time limit set by the instructor.

Supplies: Document to be mailed, window envelope.

Notes to the Student:

_____

_____

_____

_____

_____

_____

Skills Assessment Requirements

Read and familiarize yourself with the procedure; complete the minimum practice requirements (MPRs). Document each MPR using proper charting technique. Complete each procedure within a reasonable amount of time, with a minimum of 85 percent accuracy.

© 2015 Pearson Education, Inc.

POINT VALUE ◆ = 3–6 points ★ = 7–9 points		PRACTICE TRIAL	GRADED TRIAL #1	GRADED TRIAL #2	NOTES:
1. ◆	Locate the mailing address on the document.				
2. ◆	Compare the location of the mailing address to the location of the window on the envelope.				
3. ★	Fold the document so that the mailing address will be viewable through the envelope's window once the document has been inserted in the envelope.				
4. ◆	Insert the document in the envelope.				
5. ★	Verify that the address is viewable through the window.				
6. ◆	Seal the envelope.				

© 2015 Pearson Education, Inc.

Name: _____

Date: _____

Document: Enter the appropriate information in the chart below.

Grading

Points Earned	_____		
Points Possible	_____	42	42
Percent Grade (Points Earned/Points Possible)	_____		
PASS:	_____	❏ YES ❏ NO ❏ N/A	❏ YES ❏ NO ❏ N/A

Instructor Sign-Off

Instructor: _____ **Date:** _____

© 2015 Pearson Education, Inc.

Procedure 7-6:

Open and Sort Mail

Objective: Open and sort the office mail correctly within the time limit set by the instructor.

Supplies: A stack of incoming mail, including payments from insurance companies and patients, advertisements, drug samples, magazines, professional journals, bills for office services, a letter to the physician marked "Personal and Confidential," and consultation reports from other physicians; date stamp; letter opener.

Affective Behaviors: Affective behaviors provide a professional approach to a skill that enhances the patient encounter. These behaviors may also display sensitivity to patients' rights, enhance communication, convey an understanding of laws and regulations, and/or provide an overall professional component to the medical assisting profession. Pay close attention to these skills, which appear in **_bold, italicized_** font.

Notes to the Student:

_____
_____
_____
_____
_____
_____
_____

Skills Assessment Requirements

Read and familiarize yourself with the procedure; complete the minimum practice requirements (MPRs). Document each MPR using proper charting technique. Complete each procedure within a reasonable amount of time, with a minimum of 85 percent accuracy.

© 2015 Pearson Education, Inc.

POINT VALUE ◆ = 3–6 points ★ = 7–9 points		PRACTICE TRIAL	GRADED TRIAL #1	GRADED TRIAL #2	NOTES:
1. ◆	Using a date stamp, stamp the date on each received item.				
2. ★	**Remember information contained in the mail may be regarding patient care, and patient privacy must be respected.** Sort the mail into the appropriate files according to the following: • Physician—Correspondence from other physicians, hospitals, or laboratories, as well as any professional journals • Office manager—Bills for office services, drug samples, advertisements for supplies or services • Receptionist—Magazines • Billing office—Payments from patients or insurance companies, correspondence from insurance companies				
3. ◆	Open each piece of mail, except for the piece marked "Personal and Confidential."				
4. ◆	Distribute the mail appropriately. Leave the mail piece marked "Personal and Confidential" on the physician's desk.				

© 2015 Pearson Education, Inc.

Name: _____

Date: _____

Document: Enter the appropriate information in the chart below.

Grading

Points Earned	_____		
Points Possible	_____	27	27
Percent Grade (Points Earned/Points Possible)	_____		
PASS:	_____	❏ YES ❏ NO ❏ N/A	❏ YES ❏ NO ❏ N/A

Instructor Sign-Off

Instructor: _____ **Date:** _____

© 2015 Pearson Education, Inc.

Name: _____

Date: _____

Procedure 7-7:

Annotate Written Correspondence

Objective: Annotate written correspondence correctly within the time limit set by the instructor.

Supplies: Written correspondence, highlighter pen, letter opener.

Notes to the Student:

_____

_____

_____

_____

_____

_____

_____

Skills Assessment Requirements

Read and familiarize yourself with the procedure; complete the minimum practice requirements (MPRs). Document each MPR using proper charting technique. Complete each procedure within a reasonable amount of time, with a minimum of 85 percent accuracy.

© 2015 Pearson Education, Inc.

Name: _____

Date: _____

POINT VALUE ◆ = 3–6 points ★ = 7–9 points		PRACTICE TRIAL	GRADED TRIAL #1	GRADED TRIAL #2	NOTES:
1. ◆	Open the envelope with the document to be annotated.				
2. ◆	Read the document once in its entirety.				
3. ★	Using the highlighter pen, review the document again, highlighting such pertinent information as: • Patient's name • Findings of any examination or laboratory work • Dates for followup appointments • Diagnosis				
4. ★	Read the document a third time to ensure all pertinent information has been noted.				
5. ◆	Place the annotated document on the physician's desk for review.				

© 2015 Pearson Education, Inc.

Name: _____

Date: _____

Document: Enter the appropriate information in the chart below.

Grading

Points Earned	_____		
Points Possible	_____	42	42
Percent Grade (Points Earned/Points Possible)	_____		
PASS:	_____	❏ YES ❏ NO ❏ N/A	❏ YES ❏ NO ❏ N/A

Instructor Sign-Off

Instructor: _____ **Date:** _____

© 2015 Pearson Education, Inc.

Name: _____

Date: _____

Procedure 8-1:

Answer the Telephone in a Professional Manner

Objective: Answer the medical office telephone correctly within the time limit set by the instructor.

Supplies: Pen, paper, telephone.

Affective Behaviors: Affective behaviors provide a professional approach to a skill that enhances the patient encounter. These behaviors may also display sensitivity to patients' rights, enhance communication, convey an understanding of laws and regulations, and/or provide an overall professional component to the medical assisting profession. Pay close attention to these skills, which appear in ***bold, italicized*** font.

Notes to the Student:

_____

_____

_____

_____

_____

_____

Skills Assessment Requirements

Read and familiarize yourself with the procedure; complete the minimum practice requirements (MPRs). Document each MPR using proper charting technique. Complete each procedure within a reasonable amount of time, with a minimum of 85 percent accuracy.

© 2015 Pearson Education, Inc.

Name: _____

Date: _____

POINT VALUE ◆ = 3–6 points ★ = 7–9 points		PRACTICE TRIAL	GRADED TRIAL #1	GRADED TRIAL #2	NOTES:
1. ★	**Smile** as you answer the telephone; **answer it between the second and third rings.**				
2. ◆	State the office's name, followed by your name.				
3. ◆	If the caller fails to provide a personal name, ask for it and write it down.				
4. ◆	Determine the reason for the call.				
5. ◆	If the caller is having a medical emergency, ask if someone in the medical office might come to the phone to speak to the caller about it. If not, motion a coworker to dial for emergency services while keeping the patient on the line.				
6. ◆	If the patient is calling to speak with another member of the health care team, transfer the call to that person if available.				
7. ★	When a requested party is unavailable, record a message. Include the name of the caller, the date and time of the call, the telephone number where the caller can be reached, the reason for the call, and the name of the person the caller wishes to reach.				
8. ◆	When taking a message, inform the caller when the call will likely be returned.				

© 2015 Pearson Education, Inc.

9. ◆	Clarify information (e.g., appointment time) as appropriate.				
10. ◆	**End the call by asking, "Is there anything else I can do for you?" and then by saying, "Thank you and have a nice day."** Allow the caller to hang up before hanging up.				
11. ◆	Route any message to the proper staff member.				
12. ★	Chart any health care-related information into the patient's chart as appropriate.				

© 2015 Pearson Education, Inc.

Name: _____

Date: _____

Document: Enter the appropriate information in the chart below.

Grading

Points Earned	_____		
Points Possible	_____	81	81
Percent Grade (Points Earned/Points Possible)	_____		
PASS:	_____	❏ YES ❏ NO ❏ N/A	❏ YES ❏ NO ❏ N/A

Instructor Sign-Off

Instructor: _____ **Date:** _____

© 2015 Pearson Education, Inc.

Name: _____

Date: _____

Procedure 8-2:

Take a Telephone Message

Objective: Take a message correctly within the time limit set by the instructor.

Supplies: Pen, telephone message pad or electronic message system, telephone.

Affective Behaviors: Affective behaviors provide a professional approach to a skill that enhances the patient encounter. These behaviors may also display sensitivity to patients' rights, enhance communication, convey an understanding of laws and regulations, and/or provide an overall professional component to the medical assisting profession. Pay close attention to these skills, which appear in **_bold, italicized_** font.

Notes to the Student:

_____

_____

_____

_____

_____

_____

Skills Assessment Requirements

Read and familiarize yourself with the procedure; complete the minimum practice requirements (MPRs). Document each MPR using proper charting technique. Complete each procedure within a reasonable amount of time, with a minimum of 85 percent accuracy.

© 2015 Pearson Education, Inc.

Name: _____

Date: _____

POINT VALUE ◆ = 3–6 points ★ = 7–9 points		PRACTICE TRIAL	GRADED TRIAL #1	GRADED TRIAL #2	NOTES:
1. ★	**Smile and answer the telephone call by the second ring.**				
2. ◆	Once the caller identifies the desired party, reach for the message pad.				
3. ◆	Ask for the caller's full name, verify the spelling, and document it on the pad.				
4. ◆	Verify the name of the party the caller is trying to reach, and document it manually or electronically.				
5. ◆	Ask for the reason for the call, and document it manually or electronically.				
6. ◆	Ask for the caller's telephone number, including area code, and document it manually or electronically.				
7. ◆	**Repeat the telephone number to the caller to verify it was documented correctly.**				
8. ◆	Document the date and time of the call manually or electronically.				
9. ◆	Document your name or initials manually or electronically.				
10. ◆	**Tell the caller when to expect a return call.**				
11. ★	**Ask if there is anything you can do for the caller, say thank you, and then good-bye. Allow the caller to hang up first.**				
12. ◆	Route the message to its intended recipient.				

© 2015 Pearson Education, Inc.

Name: _____

Date: _____

Document: Enter the appropriate information in the chart below.

Grading

Points Earned	_____		
Points Possible	_____	78	78
Percent Grade (Points Earned/Points Possible)	_____		
PASS:	_____	❏ YES ❏ NO ❏ N/A	❏ YES ❏ NO ❏ N/A

Instructor Sign-Off

Instructor: _____   **Date:** _____

© 2015 Pearson Education, Inc.

Name: _____

Date: _____

Procedure 8-3:

Call a Pharmacy with Prescription Orders

Objective: Call a pharmacy with a new or refill prescription order within the time limit set by the instructor.

Supplies: Telephone, patient's chart, pen, prescription information, pharmacy telephone number.

Affective Behaviors: Affective behaviors provide a professional approach to a skill that enhances the patient encounter. These behaviors may also display sensitivity to patients' rights, enhance communication, convey an understanding of laws and regulations, and/or provide an overall professional component to the medical assisting profession. Pay close attention to these skills, which appear in **bold, *italicized*** font.

Notes to the Student:

_____

_____

_____

_____

_____

_____

Skills Assessment Requirements

Read and familiarize yourself with the procedure; complete the minimum practice requirements (MPRs). Document each MPR using proper charting technique. Complete each procedure within a reasonable amount of time, with a minimum of 85 percent accuracy.

© 2015 Pearson Education, Inc.

Name: _____

Date: _____

POINT VALUE ◆ = 3–6 points ★ = 7–9 points		PRACTICE TRIAL	GRADED TRIAL #1	GRADED TRIAL #2	NOTES:
1. ◆	Carefully read the prescription the physician has ordered.				
2. ★	**Ask the physician any questions about the prescription if needed.**				
3. ◆	Call the pharmacy where the patient would like the prescription filled.				
4. ◆	Give the pharmacist the patient's name, and **verify the spelling.**				
5. ◆	Give the pharmacist the patient's birthdate.				
6. ◆	Give the pharmacist the medication's name, dosage, and directions per the physician. Alert the pharmacist to any drug allergies the patient has.				
7. ★	**Ask the pharmacist to repeat the information for verification**, and inform the pharmacist if the patient is en route to the pharmacy.				
8. ★	Document the prescription, including pharmacy name and telephone number, on the medication record in the patient's medical chart.				

© 2015 Pearson Education, Inc.

Name: _____

Date: _____

Document: Enter the appropriate information in the chart below.

Grading

Points Earned	_____		
Points Possible	_____	57	57
Percent Grade (Points Earned/Points Possible)	_____		
PASS:	_____	❑ YES ❑ NO ❑ N/A	❑ YES ❑ NO ❑ N/A

Instructor Sign-Off

Instructor: _____   **Date:** _____

© 2015 Pearson Education, Inc.

Procedure 9-1:

Open the Office

Objective: Open the medical office correctly within the time limit set by the instructor.

Supplies: Checklist of office opening procedures.

Affective Behaviors: Affective behaviors provide a professional approach to a skill that enhances the patient encounter. These behaviors may also display sensitivity to patients' rights, enhance communication, convey an understanding of laws and regulations, and/or provide an overall professional component to the medical assisting profession. Pay close attention to these skills, which appear in ***bold, italicized*** font.

Notes to the Student:

_____

_____

_____

_____

_____

_____

_____

Skills Assessment Requirements

Read and familiarize yourself with the procedure; complete the minimum practice requirements (MPRs). Document each MPR using proper charting technique. Complete each procedure within a reasonable amount of time, with a minimum of 85 percent accuracy.

© 2015 Pearson Education, Inc.

POINT VALUE ◆ = 3–6 points ★ = 7–9 points		PRACTICE TRIAL	GRADED TRIAL #1	GRADED TRIAL #2	NOTES:
1. ★	**Arrive in the office at least 30 minutes before the first patient appointment.**				
2. ◆	Turn off the office alarm system.				
3. ◆	Turn on all appropriate lights and equipment.				
4. ◆	Retrieve messages from the office answering system, and return telephone calls as appropriate.				
5. ◆	Verify that all patient charts needed for the morning were pulled last night and that all needed information is attached to those charts.				
6. ◆	Check the office for **safety and cleanliness**. For example, be sure all garbage cans are empty.				
7. ◆	When the office is ready, unlock the door for patients to enter.				

© 2015 Pearson Education, Inc.

Name: _____

Date: _____

Document: Enter the appropriate information in the chart below.

Grading

Points Earned	_____		
Points Possible	_____	45	45
Percent Grade (Points Earned/Points Possible)	_____		
PASS:	_____	❑ YES ❑ NO ❑ N/A	❑ YES ❑ NO ❑ N/A

Instructor Sign-Off

Instructor: _____ Date: _____

© 2015 Pearson Education, Inc.

Procedure 9-2:

Greet and Register Patients

Objective: Correctly greet and register patients.

Supplies: Patient history form, pen, clipboard.

Affective Behaviors: Affective behaviors provide a professional approach to a skill that enhances the patient encounter. These behaviors may also display sensitivity to patients' rights, enhance communication, convey an understanding of laws and regulations, and/or provide an overall professional component to the medical assisting profession. Pay close attention to these skills, which appear in **bold, *italicized*** font.

Notes to the Student:

_____

_____

_____

_____

_____

_____

_____

Skills Assessment Requirements

Read and familiarize yourself with the procedure; complete the minimum practice requirements (MPRs). Document each MPR using proper charting technique. Complete each procedure within a reasonable amount of time, with a minimum of 85 percent accuracy.

© 2015 Pearson Education, Inc.

Name: _____

Date: _____

POINT VALUE ◆ = 3–6 points ★ = 7–9 points		PRACTICE TRIAL	GRADED TRIAL #1	GRADED TRIAL #2	NOTES:
1. ★	As the patient arrives at the front desk, look up and **make eye contact right away**. If you are on the telephone, **make a motion to the patient with your index finger to indicate that you will be with the patient in one moment**. If you are not on the telephone, **smile and ask the patient for her name**.				
2. ◆	Once you have obtained the patient's name, check the appointment schedule to verify the patient is there at the right time and to verify the type of appointment the patient is scheduled to have.				
3. ◆	If the patient is new to the office, give her the appropriate new patient forms to fill out on a clipboard, along with a pen.				
4. ◆	Ask the patient to take a seat in the reception area and provide the patient with an approximate amount of time that she can expect to wait before being taken back to see the provider.				
5. ★	Alert the clinical medical assistant of the patient's arrival.				

© 2015 Pearson Education, Inc.

Name: _____

Date: _____

Document: Enter the appropriate information in the chart below.

Grading

Points Earned	_____		
Points Possible	_____	36	36
Percent Grade (Points Earned/Points Possible)	_____		
PASS:	_____	❏ YES ❏ NO ❏ N/A	❏ YES ❏ NO ❏ N/A

Instructor Sign-Off

Instructor: _____ **Date:** _____

© 2015 Pearson Education, Inc.

Procedure 9-3:

Collect Payments at the Front Desk

Objective: Correctly collect payments at the front desk.

Supplies: Pen, cash receipt book, credit card machine, check endorsement stamp.

Affective Behaviors: Affective behaviors provide a professional approach to a skill that enhances the patient encounter. These behaviors may also display sensitivity to patients' rights, enhance communication, convey an understanding of laws and regulations, and/or provide an overall professional component to the medical assisting profession. Pay close attention to these skills, which appear in **_bold, italicized_** font.

Notes to the Student:

_____

_____

_____

_____

_____

_____

_____

Skills Assessment Requirements

Read and familiarize yourself with the procedure; complete the minimum practice requirements (MPRs). Document each MPR using proper charting technique. Complete each procedure within a reasonable amount of time, with a minimum of 85 percent accuracy.

© 2015 Pearson Education, Inc.

Name: _____

Date: _____

POINT VALUE ◆ = 3–6 points ★ = 7–9 points	PRACTICE TRIAL	GRADED TRIAL #1	GRADED TRIAL #2	NOTES:
1. ★ As the patient arrives at the front desk, check the computer or chart to verify the patient's copayment amount.				
2. ◆ After registering the patient, let the patient know the amount of the expected payment.				
3. ◆ Ask the patient if he would prefer to make the payment via cash, check, or credit card. *If the patient does not have the copayment, approach the matter in a sensitive manner while politely explaining the office policy regarding payment at time of service.*				
4. ◆ If the patient pays via cash, write a receipt from the cash receipt book.				
5. ◆ If the patient pays via check, endorse the check with the bank endorsement stamp. Ask the patient if he would like a written receipt. If so, write a receipt from the cash receipt book.				
6. ◆ If the patient pays via credit card, process the credit card on the credit card machine, have the patient sign the slip, and provide the patient with his portion as a receipt.				

© 2015 Pearson Education, Inc.

Name: _____

Date: _____

Document: Enter the appropriate information in the chart below.

Grading

Points Earned	_____		
Points Possible	_____	39	39
Percent Grade (Points Earned/Points Possible)	_____		
PASS:	_____	❑ YES ❑ NO ❑ N/A	❑ YES ❑ NO ❑ N/A

Instructor Sign-Off

Instructor: _____ **Date:** _____

© 2015 Pearson Education, Inc.

Procedure 9-4:

Close the Office

Objective: Close the medical office correctly within the time limit set by the instructor.

Supplies: Checklist of office closing procedures.

Affective Behaviors: Affective behaviors provide a professional approach to a skill that enhances the patient encounter. These behaviors may also display sensitivity to patients' rights, enhance communication, convey an understanding of laws and regulations, and/or provide an overall professional component to the medical assisting profession. Pay close attention to these skills, which appear in **bold, *italicized*** font.

Notes to the Student:

_____

_____

_____

_____

_____

_____

_____

Skills Assessment Requirements

Read and familiarize yourself with the procedure; complete the minimum practice requirements (MPRs). Document each MPR using proper charting technique. Complete each procedure within a reasonable amount of time, with a minimum of 85 percent accuracy.

© 2015 Pearson Education, Inc.

Name: _____

Date: _____

POINT VALUE ◆ = 3–6 points ★ = 7–9 points		PRACTICE TRIAL	GRADED TRIAL #1	GRADED TRIAL #2	NOTES:
1. ◆	Ensure all patients have exited the office. Check treatment rooms and restrooms.				
2. ◆	Verify that all the day's patient files have been routed to the appropriate area (e.g., billing, physician, clinical medical assistant).				
3. ◆	Pull all files for patients scheduled for the following morning.				
4. ★	Confirm that all information needed for the morning's patients (e.g., lab reports or consultations) is available. *Take time to locate information that is not readily available.*				
5. ◆	Attach needed information to patient files.				
6. ◆	Call to confirm any patient appointments made prior to a couple of days ago. *Be certain to follow HIPAA guidelines regarding patient privacy.*				
7. ★	Forward the telephones over to the answering system.				
8. ◆	Turn off all appropriate equipment and lights.				
9. ★	Activate the alarm and lock the doors when leaving the building.				

© 2015 Pearson Education, Inc.

Name: _____

Date: _____

Document: Enter the appropriate information in the chart below.

Grading

Points Earned	_____		
Points Possible	_____	63	63
Percent Grade (Points Earned/Points Possible)	_____		
PASS:	_____	❏ YES ❏ NO ❏ N/A	❏ YES ❏ NO ❏ N/A

Instructor Sign-Off

Instructor: _____ **Date:** _____

© 2015 Pearson Education, Inc.

Procedure 10-1:

Establish an Appointment Matrix

Objective: Correctly establish an appointment matrix.

Supplies: Pen, paper or electronic appointment schedule.

Notes to the Student:

_____

_____

_____

_____

_____

_____

_____

Skills Assessment Requirements

Read and familiarize yourself with the procedure; complete the minimum practice requirements (MPRs). Document each MPR using proper charting technique. Complete each procedure within a reasonable amount of time, with a minimum of 85 percent accuracy.

Name: _____

Date: _____

POINT VALUE ◆ = 3–6 points ★ = 7–9 points		PRACTICE TRIAL	GRADED TRIAL #1	GRADED TRIAL #2	NOTES:
1. ◆	Determine the amount of time the providers want patients to have for each appointment type.				
2. ★	Within the appointment book, block out the time when the providers will be out of the office for lunch or other appointments. If using an electronic scheduling system, block out the time in the electronic appointment schedule.				
3. ★	Highlight or create blocks of time in the appointment book for appointments the provider specifies as those he would only like a limited number of, such as physical exams. If using an electronic appointment system, use the features contained within the program to accomplish this task.				
4. ◆	Go over the created appointment matrix with the providers to determine where any adjustments need to be made.				

© 2015 Pearson Education, Inc.

Name: _____

Date: _____

Document: Enter the appropriate information in the chart below.

Grading

Points Earned	_____		
Points Possible	_____	30	30
Percent Grade (Points Earned/Points Possible)	_____		
PASS:	_____	❑ YES ❑ NO ❑ N/A	❑ YES ❑ NO ❑ N/A

Instructor Sign-Off

Instructor: _____ **Date:** _____

Procedure 10-2:

Schedule a New Patient Appointment

Objective: Correctly schedule a new patient who calls the medical office.

Supplies: Telephone, blue or black ink pen, paper or electronic appointment book, new patient checklist.

Affective Behaviors: Affective behaviors provide a professional approach to a skill that enhances the patient encounter. These behaviors may also display sensitivity to patients' rights, enhance communication, convey an understanding of laws and regulations, and/or provide an overall professional component to the medical assisting profession. Pay close attention to these skills, which appear in **_bold, italicized_** font.

Notes to the Student:

_____

_____

_____

_____

_____

_____

_____

Skills Assessment Requirements

Read and familiarize yourself with the procedure; complete the minimum practice requirements (MPRs). Document each MPR using proper charting technique. Complete each procedure within a reasonable amount of time, with a minimum of 85 percent accuracy.

© 2015 Pearson Education, Inc.

Name: _____

Date: _____

POINT VALUE ◆ = 3–6 points ★ = 7–9 points		PRACTICE TRIAL	GRADED TRIAL #1	GRADED TRIAL #2	NOTES:
1. ◆	Using a **professional, friendly voice, smile and answer the telephone by the second ring**.				
2. ◆	State the office name, followed by your name.				
3. ◆	When the caller does not self-identify as a new patient, ask the caller the date of his or her last visit in the office. If the patient states she has not been seen previously, the medical assistant may proceed with scheduling the patient as a new patient.				
4. ◆	Ask the patient to spell her first and last names.				
5. ◆	Write the patient's full name on the paper.				
6. ◆	Ask the patient for work and home telephone numbers, and for home address.				
7. ◆	Ask the patient how she was referred to the office.				
8. ◆	Ask the patient to identify the type of health insurance that she will be using.				
9. ★	Confirm that your physician participates in the patient's health care plan.				
10. ◆	If the physician does not participate in the patient's health plan, advise the patient that she may fail to receive preferred benefits or may need to pay in full for services.				

© 2015 Pearson Education, Inc.

Name: _____

Date: _____

11. ◆	Ask the patient to state the condition prompting the visit.				
12. ◆	Ask the patient to define the length of the condition.				
13. ◆	Offer the patient appointment times to see the physician.				
14. ★	Schedule the patient.				
15. ◆	If mailing paperwork to the patient to complete before the appointment, direct the patient to complete the paperwork before the visit.				
16. ◆	If the patient will need to complete the paperwork at the first visit, direct her to arrive 15 minutes before the appointment's scheduled start time. In offices that keep electronic versions of their medical forms online, assistants will direct patients on how to fill out the paperwork prior to their visit.				
17. ◆	Document the patient's information in the manual or electronic appointment schedule.				
18. ◆	Ask the patient if directions to the office are needed.				
19. ◆	Give the patient any needed parking information.				
20. ★	Confirm the appointment date and time with the patient. **Thank the patient for calling and ask if there is anything else you can do for her.**				
21. ◆	**Allow the patient to hang up the telephone before hanging up yourself.**				

Document: Enter the appropriate information in the chart below.

Grading

Points Earned	_____		
Points Possible	_____	135	135
Percent Grade (Points Earned/Points Possible)	_____		
PASS:	_____	❏ YES ❏ NO ❏ N/A	❏ YES ❏ NO ❏ N/A

Instructor Sign-Off

Instructor: _____ **Date:** _____

© 2015 Pearson Education, Inc.

Name: _____

Date: _____

Procedure 10-3:

Schedule an Established Patient Appointment

Objective: Schedule a patient appointment correctly within the time limit set by the instructor.

Supplies: Paper or electronic appointment schedule, blue or black ink pen, patient's chart.

Affective Behaviors: Affective behaviors provide a professional approach to a skill that enhances the patient encounter. These behaviors may also display sensitivity to patients' rights, enhance communication, convey an understanding of laws and regulations, and/or provide an overall professional component to the medical assisting profession. Pay close attention to these skills, which appear in **_bold, italicized_** font.

Notes to the Student:

_____

_____

_____

_____

_____

_____

Skills Assessment Requirements

Read and familiarize yourself with the procedure; complete the minimum practice requirements (MPRs). Document each MPR using proper charting technique. Complete each procedure within a reasonable amount of time, with a minimum of 85 percent accuracy.

© 2015 Pearson Education, Inc.

Name: _____

Date: _____

POINT VALUE ◆ = 3–6 points ★ = 7–9 points		PRACTICE TRIAL	GRADED TRIAL #1	GRADED TRIAL #2	NOTES:
1. ★	***Using a professional, friendly voice, smile and answer the telephone by the second ring.***				
2. ◆	Locate the chart of the patient to be scheduled.				
3. ◆	Determine the type of appointment that is needed.				
4. ◆	Determine the patient's schedule.				
5. ◆	Determine the physician's schedule.				
6. ◆	Enter the patient in the appointment schedule.				
7. ★	Restate the appointment date and time to the patient. If the patient is in the office, provide a written reminder card. Remind the patient to bring any needed items to the appointment or to follow any procedures (e.g., fasting before the visit). ***If the patient called on the phone, thank the patient for calling and ask if there is anything else you can do for him.***				

© 2015 Pearson Education, Inc.

Name: _____

Date: _____

Document: Enter the appropriate information in the chart below.

Grading

Points Earned	_____		
Points Possible	_____	48	48
Percent Grade (Points Earned/Points Possible)	_____		
PASS:	_____	❑ YES ❑ NO ❑ N/A	❑ YES ❑ NO ❑ N/A

Instructor Sign-Off

Instructor: _____ **Date:** _____

© 2015 Pearson Education, Inc.

Name: _____

Date: _____

Procedure 10-4:

Use Patient Reminder Cards

Objective: Correctly use patient reminder cards.

Supplies: Pen, paper or electronic appointment book, appointment reminder card.

Affective Behaviors: Affective behaviors provide a professional approach to a skill that enhances the patient encounter. These behaviors may also display sensitivity to patients' rights, enhance communication, convey an understanding of laws and regulations, and/or provide an overall professional component to the medical assisting profession. Pay close attention to these skills, which appear in **bold, italicized** font.

Notes to the Student:

_____

_____

_____

_____

_____

_____

Skills Assessment Requirements

Read and familiarize yourself with the procedure; complete the minimum practice requirements (MPRs). Document each MPR using proper charting technique. Complete each procedure within a reasonable amount of time, with a minimum of 85 percent accuracy.

© 2015 Pearson Education, Inc.

Name: _____

Date: _____

POINT VALUE ◆ = 3–6 points ★ = 7–9 points		PRACTICE TRIAL	GRADED TRIAL #1	GRADED TRIAL #2	NOTES:
1. ◆	As the patient arrives at the reception desk, look at the fee slip to verify when the provider wants the patient to return for an appointment.				
2. ◆	Ask the patient if there is a day or time that works best for his schedule for the appointment.				
3. ◆	Check the appointment book to find an appointment time that fits with the patient's schedule.				
4. ◆	After verifying that the appointment will work with the patient's schedule, write or type the appointment into the appointment schedule.				
5. ★	Write the patient's appointment on a reminder card and give the card to the patient. ***Thank the patient for visiting the office and bid the patient a good day.***				

© 2015 Pearson Education, Inc.

Name: _____

Date: _____

Document: Enter the appropriate information in the chart below.

Grading

Points Earned	_____		
Points Possible	_____	33	33
Percent Grade (Points Earned/Points Possible)	_____		
PASS:	_____	❏ YES ❏ NO ❏ N/A	❏ YES ❏ NO ❏ N/A

Instructor Sign-Off

Instructor: _____ **Date:** _____

© 2015 Pearson Education, Inc.

Procedure 10-5:

Reschedule a Missed Patient Appointment

Objective: Reschedule a missed patient appointment correctly within the time limit set by the instructor.

Supplies: Paper or electronic appointment schedule, blue or black ink pen, patient's chart.

Affective Behaviors: Affective behaviors provide a professional approach to a skill that enhances the patient encounter. These behaviors may also display sensitivity to patients' rights, enhance communication, convey an understanding of laws and regulations, and/or provide an overall professional component to the medical assisting profession. Pay close attention to these skills, which appear in **_bold, italicized_** font.

Notes to the Student:

_____

_____

_____

_____

_____

_____

_____

Skills Assessment Requirements

Read and familiarize yourself with the procedure; complete the minimum practice requirements (MPRs). Document each MPR using proper charting technique. Complete each procedure within a reasonable amount of time, with a minimum of 85 percent accuracy.

© 2015 Pearson Education, Inc.

Name: _____

Date: _____

POINT VALUE ◆ = 3–6 points ★ = 7–9 points		PRACTICE TRIAL	GRADED TRIAL #1	GRADED TRIAL #2	NOTES:
1. ◆	**Fifteen minutes after the patient's appointment time, call the patient's home telephone number.**				
2. ★	If the patient answers: • Point out the missed appointment time and **politely ask for an appropriate time to reschedule.** • If the patient reschedules the appointment, document the new appointment in the appointment book as well as the patient's chart. Also chart that the patient missed the originally scheduled appointment. • If the patient does not wish to reschedule, **politely state that you will inform the physician.** Chart the missed appointment and refusal to reschedule in the patient's chart, and give the chart to the physician.				
3. ★	If the patient fails to answer: • Leave a message on voice mail or with the person who answers. **Be certain not to disclose confidential patient information.** An appropriate message is "This is state your name at state the physician's name. We had you scheduled for an appointment today at state time, and I'm calling to reschedule. Please call me back at state telephone number." • In the patient's chart document the missed appointment and the message.				

© 2015 Pearson Education, Inc.

Document: Enter the appropriate information in the chart below.

Grading

Points Earned	_____		
Points Possible	_____	24	24
Percent Grade (Points Earned/Points Possible)	_____		
PASS:	_____	❏ YES ❏ NO ❏ N/A	❏ YES ❏ NO ❏ N/A

Instructor Sign-Off

Instructor: _____ **Date:** _____

© 2015 Pearson Education, Inc.

Name: _____

Date: _____

Procedure 10-6:

Manage the Physician's Professional Schedule and Travel

Objective: Manage the physician's professional schedule and travel correctly within the time limit set by the instructor.

Supplies: A telephone; a list of the physician's travel needs, including dates and times of the meeting or seminar, place of the seminar, and physician preference for airline and hotel arrangements; paper and a pen.

Notes to the Student:

_____

_____

_____

_____

_____

_____

_____

Skills Assessment Requirements

Read and familiarize yourself with the procedure; complete the minimum practice requirements (MPRs). Document each MPR using proper charting technique. Complete each procedure within a reasonable amount of time, with a minimum of 85 percent accuracy.

© 2015 Pearson Education, Inc.

Name: _____

Date: _____

POINT VALUE ◆ = 3–6 points ★ = 7–9 points	PRACTICE TRIAL	GRADED TRIAL #1	GRADED TRIAL #2	NOTES:
1. ◆ Call the physician's preferred airline and book the appropriate flight.				
2. ★ Make a note of the date, time, airline, and flight number for both departure time and arrival time for both the outgoing flight and the return flight.				
3. ◆ Call the physician's preferred hotel and book the appropriate room.				
4. ★ Make a note of the confirmation number for the hotel room.				
5. ◆ Arrange for any necessary transportation to or from the hotel and airport.				
6. ◆ Create a list of all arrangements made and give the list to the physician.				
7. ◆ Give a copy of the list of arrangements to the office manager and to the receptionist.				
8. ★ Verify the receptionist has blocked out the dates the physician will be away, if applicable.				

© 2015 Pearson Education, Inc.

Name: _____

Date: _____

Document: Enter the appropriate information in the chart below.

Grading

Points Earned	_____		
Points Possible	_____	57	57
Percent Grade (Points Earned/Points Possible)	_____		
PASS:	_____	❏ YES ❏ NO ❏ N/A	❏ YES ❏ NO ❏ N/A

Instructor Sign-Off

Instructor: _____ **Date:** _____

© 2015 Pearson Education, Inc.

Procedure 10-7:

Schedule a Hospital Procedure

Objective: Schedule a hospital procedure correctly within the time limit set by the instructor.

Supplies: Patient's chart, hospital/surgery scheduling form, scheduling guidelines, calendar, telephone, notepad, pen.

Affective Behaviors: Affective behaviors provide a professional approach to a skill that enhances the patient encounter. These behaviors may also display sensitivity to patients' rights, enhance communication, convey an understanding of laws and regulations, and/or provide an overall professional component to the medical assisting profession. Pay close attention to these skills, which appear in **_bold, italicized_** font.

Notes to the Student:

_____

_____

_____

_____

_____

_____

Skills Assessment Requirements

Read and familiarize yourself with the procedure; complete the minimum practice requirements (MPRs). Document each MPR using proper charting technique. Complete each procedure within a reasonable amount of time, with a minimum of 85 percent accuracy.

© 2015 Pearson Education, Inc.

Name: _____

Date: _____

POINT VALUE ◆ = 3–6 points ★ = 7–9 points		PRACTICE TRIAL	GRADED TRIAL #1	GRADED TRIAL #2	NOTES:
1. ◆	Obtain information from the physician or clinical medical assistant about the needed surgery or procedure and the desired hospital.				
2. ◆	Call the patient's insurance carrier to obtain preauthorization for the procedure.				
3. ★	Document the preauthorization number in the patient's chart along with the name of the customer service representative spoken to at the insurance company.				
4. ◆	If the patient is in the clinic, ask what date or time would be most convenient for the procedure. If the patient is not in the clinic, call the patient to determine scheduling needs.				
5. ◆	Call the hospital to communicate the procedure the physician has planned, the time needed for the procedure, and the date preferred for the procedure.				
6. ★	Provide the hospital staff the patient's information, including name, birthdate, address, telephone number, insurance information, and preauthorization number. Also relay all pertinent information, such as allergies or disabilities. **Only provide the hospital with the necessary patient information.**				

© 2015 Pearson Education, Inc.

7. ◆	After agreeing on a date and time, give the information to the patient and enter it in the physician's appointment schedule.				
8. ◆	Advise the patient that the hospital will likely call to provide instructions and verify the check-in date and time.				
9. ◆	Schedule the patient for a postoperative appointment in the physician's office, if needed.				
10. ★	Chart all information in the patient's medical record, and give the chart to the physician for review.				

Document: Enter the appropriate information in the chart below.

Grading

Points Earned	_____		
Points Possible	_____	69	69
Percent Grade (Points Earned/Points Possible)	_____		
PASS:	_____	❏ YES ❏ NO ❏ N/A	❏ YES ❏ NO ❏ N/A

Instructor Sign-Off

Instructor: _____ **Date:** _____

© 2015 Pearson Education, Inc.

Name: _____

Date: _____

Procedure 10-8:

Schedule an Inpatient Admission

Objective: Schedule an inpatient admission correctly within the time limit set by the instructor.

Supplies: Patient's chart, inpatient scheduling guidelines, calendar, telephone, notepad, pen.

Affective Behaviors: Affective behaviors provide a professional approach to a skill that enhances the patient encounter. These behaviors may also display sensitivity to patients' rights, enhance communication, convey an understanding of laws and regulations, and/or provide an overall professional component to the medical assisting profession. Pay close attention to these skills, which appear in **bold, italicized** font.

Notes to the Student:

_____

_____

_____

_____

_____

_____

_____

Skills Assessment Requirements

Read and familiarize yourself with the procedure; complete the minimum practice requirements (MPRs). Document each MPR using proper charting technique. Complete each procedure within a reasonable amount of time, with a minimum of 85 percent accuracy.

POINT VALUE ◆ = 3–6 points ★ = 7–9 points		PRACTICE TRIAL	GRADED TRIAL #1	GRADED TRIAL #2	NOTES:
1. ◆	Call the patient's insurance carrier to obtain preauthorization for the procedure, the needed followup, and the allowable number of hospital days. **Thank the insurance representative for her assistance.**				
2. ★	Document the preauthorization number in the patient's chart along with the name of the customer service representative spoken to at the insurance company.				
3. ★	Call the hospital admissions office with the patient's name, physician's name, and reason for admission.				
4. ◆	Let the admissions office know when the physician would like the patient to be admitted.				
5. ◆	Give the admissions office the patient's contact information, birthdate, insurance information, and preauthorization number.				
6. ◆	Instruct the patient when to arrive at the hospital and where to go once there.				

© 2015 Pearson Education, Inc.

7. ◆	Give the patient any specifics on what to bring (or not) to the hospital. **_Ask the patient if he has any questions that need to be answered._**				
8. ★	Chart all information in the patient's medical record, and give the chart to the physician for review.				

© 2015 Pearson Education, Inc.

Name: _____

Date: _____

Document: Enter the appropriate information in the chart below.

Grading

Points Earned	_____		
Points Possible	_____	57	57
Percent Grade (Points Earned/Points Possible)	_____		
PASS:	_____	❏ YES ❏ NO ❏ N/A	❏ YES ❏ NO ❏ N/A

Instructor Sign-Off

Instructor: _____ **Date:** _____

© 2015 Pearson Education, Inc.

Procedure 11-1:

Prepare the Medical Chart

Objective: Prepare a patient medical chart correctly within the time limit set by the instructor.

Supplies: Medical chart, metal file clips, medication record sheet, progress notes record, color-coded alphabet stickers, file label, two-hole punch, patient's name.

Notes to the Student:

_____

_____

_____

_____

_____

_____

_____

Skills Assessment Requirements

Read and familiarize yourself with the procedure; complete the minimum practice requirements (MPRs). Document each MPR using proper charting technique. Complete each procedure within a reasonable amount of time, with a minimum of 85 percent accuracy.

© 2015 Pearson Education, Inc.

Name: _____

Date: _____

POINT VALUE ◆ = 3–6 points ★ = 7–9 points		PRACTICE TRIAL	GRADED TRIAL #1	GRADED TRIAL #2	NOTES:
1. ◆	Print the patient's name on a file label, with the last name followed by first name and middle initial. For example, print "Smith, John R." on the file label.				
2. ★	Verify the spelling of the patient's name.				
3. ◆	Using the color-coded alphabet stickers, place the first two letters of the patient's last name on the file near the file label. In the preceding example, "SM" stickers would appear near the file label.				
4. ◆	One space after the stickers in the preceding step, place a color-coded alphabet sticker for the first letter of the patient's first name. Building on the preceding example for John R. Smith, the file stickers would read "SM [space] J."				
5. ◆	Add metal file clips to both sides of the file.				
6. ◆	Using the two-hole punch, punch holes in the top of the documents to be filed in the patient's chart. Punch such documents as the patient's history form, the Health Insurance Portability and Accountability Act (HIPAA) notification form, and the patient's consent to be examined.				
7. ◆	Place the medication record sheet on one side of the chart.				

© 2015 Pearson Education, Inc.

8. ◆	Place the progress report sheet on the other side of the chart.				
9. ★	On the front of the chart in red ink, note any of the patient's known allergies. When the patient has no known allergies, write "NKA" (i.e., no known allergies) on the front of the chart.				

© 2015 Pearson Education, Inc.

Name: _____

Date: _____

Document: Enter the appropriate information in the chart below.

Grading

Points Earned	_____		
Points Possible	_____	60	60
Percent Grade (Points Earned/Points Possible)	_____		
PASS:	_____	❏ YES ❏ NO ❏ N/A	❏ YES ❏ NO ❏ N/A

Instructor Sign-Off

Instructor: _____ **Date:** _____

© 2015 Pearson Education, Inc.

Procedure 11-2:

Correct Errors in the Patient Medical Record

Objective: Correct an error in the patient medical record correctly within the time limit set by the instructor.

Supplies: Patient medical record, blue or black ink pen.

Notes to the Student:

_____

_____

_____

_____

_____

_____

Skills Assessment Requirements

Read and familiarize yourself with the procedure; complete the minimum practice requirements (MPRs). Document each MPR using proper charting technique. Complete each procedure within a reasonable amount of time, with a minimum of 85 percent accuracy.

© 2015 Pearson Education, Inc.

POINT VALUE ◆ = 3–6 points ★ = 7–9 points		PRACTICE TRIAL	GRADED TRIAL #1	GRADED TRIAL #2	NOTES:
1. ◆	Locate the error in the patient's medical record.				
2. ◆	Draw a straight line through the error.				
3. ★	Initial and place the date above the line.				
4. ★	When the corrected entry will fit above the line, write the correction there. Include the date of the new entry and your initials. When the corrected entry will not fit above the line, add a new entry to the progress notes with the day's date and the word *ADDENDUM* in all capitals. Include the date of the addendum, enter the corrected entry, and initial the entry.				

© 2015 Pearson Education, Inc.

Name: _____

Date: _____

Document: Enter the appropriate information in the chart below.

Grading

Points Earned	_____		
Points Possible	_____	30	30
Percent Grade (Points Earned/Points Possible)	_____		
PASS:	_____	❏ YES ❏ NO ❏ N/A	❏ YES ❏ NO ❏ N/A

Instructor Sign-Off

Instructor: _____ **Date:** _____

© 2015 Pearson Education, Inc.

Procedure 11-3:

Chart Patient Telephone Calls

Objective: Chart a patient telephone call correctly within the time limit set by the instructor.

Supplies: Notepad and pen, paper or electronic patient medical record.

Affective Behaviors: Affective behaviors provide a professional approach to a skill that enhances the patient encounter. These behaviors may also display sensitivity to patients' rights, enhance communication, convey an understanding of laws and regulations, and/or provide an overall professional component to the medical assisting profession. Pay close attention to these skills, which appear in **_bold, italicized_** font.

Notes to the Student:

_____

_____

_____

_____

_____

_____

_____

Skills Assessment Requirements

Read and familiarize yourself with the procedure; complete the minimum practice requirements (MPRs). Document each MPR using proper charting technique. Complete each procedure within a reasonable amount of time, with a minimum of 85 percent accuracy.

© 2015 Pearson Education, Inc.

Name: _____

Date: _____

POINT VALUE ◆ = 3–6 points ★ = 7–9 points		PRACTICE TRIAL	GRADED TRIAL #1	GRADED TRIAL #2	NOTES:
1. ◆	While answering an incoming patient call, determine if the call is medically relevant to the patient's care in the office.				
2. ◆	When the call is medically relevant to the patient's care, note the call's time and date, the patient's complete name, and the nature of the message.				
3. ◆	When the call ends, bring up the chart electronically in the electronic health record or pull the patient's chart.				
4. ◆	In the progress notes section of the patient's chart, note the current date and time.				
5. ★	Enter the medically relevant portion of the call in the patient's medical record, using quotation marks to indicate any direct quotes from the patient.				
6. ◆	**Sign your name and credentials at the end of the chart entry.**				
7. ★	When the call requires the physician's attention, leave the paper chart on the physician's desk or forward the electronic message to the physician in the electronic health record. When the call does not require the physician's attention, file or close the chart.				
8. ★	After transferring all relevant information to the chart, **shred any notes from the call that contain personal patient information.**				

© 2015 Pearson Education, Inc.

Name: _____

Date: _____

Document: Enter the appropriate information in the chart below.

Grading

Points Earned	_____		
Points Possible	_____	57	57
Percent Grade (Points Earned/Points Possible)	_____		
PASS:	_____	❏ YES ❏ NO ❏ N/A	❏ YES ❏ NO ❏ N/A

Instructor Sign-Off

Instructor: _____ **Date:** _____

© 2015 Pearson Education, Inc.

Name: _____

Date: _____

Procedure 11-4:

File Documents Using the Alphabetic Filing System

Objective: Correctly file documents using the alphabetic filing system.

Supplies: Patient medical records, color-coded alphabetic file letter stickers.

Notes to the Student:

_____

_____

_____

_____

_____

_____

Skills Assessment Requirements

Read and familiarize yourself with the procedure; complete the minimum practice requirements (MPRs). Document each MPR using proper charting technique. Complete each procedure within a reasonable amount of time, with a minimum of 85 percent accuracy.

© 2015 Pearson Education, Inc.

POINT VALUE ◆ = 3–6 points ★ = 7–9 points		PRACTICE TRIAL	GRADED TRIAL #1	GRADED TRIAL #2	NOTES:
1. ◆	Using the color-coded alphabetic file letter stickers, apply stickers to each medical record using the first two letters from the patient's last name.				
2. ★	Arrange the medical records in alphabetical order by last name.				
3. ★	File the medical records accurately into the filing cabinet.				

© 2015 Pearson Education, Inc.

Name: _____

Date: _____

Document: Enter the appropriate information in the chart below.

Grading

Points Earned	_____		
Points Possible	_____	24	24
Percent Grade (Points Earned/Points Possible)	_____		
PASS:	_____	❏ YES ❏ NO ❏ N/A	❏ YES ❏ NO ❏ N/A

Instructor Sign-Off

Instructor: _____ **Date:** _____

© 2015 Pearson Education, Inc.

Name: _____

Date: _____

Procedure 11-5:

File Manually Using a Subject Filing System

Objective: Correctly file manually using a subject filing system.

Supplies: Documents to be filed by subject, alphabetic card file, index card listing subjects.

Notes to the Student:

_____

_____

_____

_____

_____

_____

_____

Skills Assessment Requirements

Read and familiarize yourself with the procedure; complete the minimum practice requirements (MPRs). Document each MPR using proper charting technique. Complete each procedure within a reasonable amount of time, with a minimum of 85 percent accuracy.

Name: _____

Date: _____

POINT VALUE ◆ = 3–6 points ★ = 7–9 points		PRACTICE TRIAL	GRADED TRIAL #1	GRADED TRIAL #2	NOTES:
1. ★	Organize the documents by subject matter.				
2. ◆	Match the subject of the document to the appropriate category on the index cards.				
3. ◆	Underline the subject title on the document.				
4. ★	File the document under the appropriate category.				
5. ◆	If the document fits into more than one category, create an index card as a cross-reference listing the name of the document and the category under which it is filed.				

© 2015 Pearson Education, Inc.

Name: _____

Date: _____

Document: Enter the appropriate information in the chart below.

Grading

Points Earned	_____		
Points Possible	_____	36	36
Percent Grade (Points Earned/Points Possible)	_____		
PASS:	_____	❏ YES ❏ NO ❏ N/A	❏ YES ❏ NO ❏ N/A

Instructor Sign-Off

Instructor: _____ **Date:** _____

© 2015 Pearson Education, Inc.

Name: _____

Date: _____

Procedure 11-6:

File Documents in Patient Medical Records

Objective: File documents into a patient's medical record correctly within the time limit set by the instructor.

Supplies: Patient medical record, documents to be filed, two-hole punch.

Notes to the Student:

_____

_____

_____

_____

_____

_____

Skills Assessment Requirements

Read and familiarize yourself with the procedure; complete the minimum practice requirements (MPRs). Document each MPR using proper charting technique. Complete each procedure within a reasonable amount of time, with a minimum of 85 percent accuracy.

© 2015 Pearson Education, Inc.

POINT VALUE ◆ = 3–6 points ★ = 7–9 points		PRACTICE TRIAL	GRADED TRIAL #1	GRADED TRIAL #2	NOTES:
1. ◆	Using the two-hole punch, punch holes in the top of each document to be filed.				
2. ★	Verify that the physician has viewed any report to be filed (e.g., laboratory or pathology report) by locating the physician's initials on the report.				
3. ★	Verify that the patient file matches the name on the documents to be filed.				
4. ◆	Using the metal clips in the file, place the documents in the patient medical record with the most recent documents on top.				
5. ◆	Fasten the metal clips.				

© 2015 Pearson Education, Inc.

Name: _____

Date: _____

Document: Enter the appropriate information in the chart below.

Grading

Points Earned	_____		
Points Possible	_____	36	36
Percent Grade (Points Earned/Points Possible)	_____		
PASS:	_____	❏ YES ❏ NO ❏ N/A	❏ YES ❏ NO ❏ N/A

Instructor Sign-Off

Instructor: _____ **Date:** _____

© 2015 Pearson Education, Inc.

Procedure 11-7:

Use the Numeric System to File the Medical Record

Objective: Correctly use the numeric system to file medical records.

Supplies: Patient medical records, color-coded numeric file stickers.

Notes to the Student:

_____

_____

_____

_____

_____

_____

Skills Assessment Requirements

Read and familiarize yourself with the procedure; complete the minimum practice requirements (MPRs). Document each MPR using proper charting technique. Complete each procedure within a reasonable amount of time, with a minimum of 85 percent accuracy.

© 2015 Pearson Education, Inc.

Name: _____

Date: _____

POINT VALUE ◆ = 3–6 points ★ = 7–9 points	PRACTICE TRIAL	GRADED TRIAL #1	GRADED TRIAL #2	NOTES:
1. ◆ Using the color-coded numeric file stickers, attach the first two numbers of the patient's medical record.				
2. ◆ After verifying that the patient's numeric identification number is accurately recorded on a master sheet kept away from the patient's files, organize the records in numeric order.				
3. ★ File the medical records in numeric order into the medical records filing system.				

© 2015 Pearson Education, Inc.

Name: _____

Date: _____

Document: Enter the appropriate information in the chart below.

Grading

Points Earned	_____		
Points Possible	_____	21	21
Percent Grade (Points Earned/Points Possible)	_____		
PASS:	_____	❏ YES ❏ NO ❏ N/A	❏ YES ❏ NO ❏ N/A

Instructor Sign-Off

Instructor: _____ **Date:** _____

© 2015 Pearson Education, Inc.

Procedure 12-1:

Correct an Electronic Health Record

Objective: Correct an electronic health record within the time limit set by the instructor.

Supplies: Computer with electronic patient medical record.

Notes to the Student:

_____

_____

_____

_____

_____

_____

_____

Skills Assessment Requirements

Read and familiarize yourself with the procedure; complete the minimum practice requirements (MPRs). Document each MPR using proper charting technique. Complete each procedure within a reasonable amount of time, with a minimum of 85 percent accuracy.

© 2015 Pearson Education, Inc.

Name: _____

Date: _____

POINT VALUE ◆ = 3–6 points ★ = 7–9 points		PRACTICE TRIAL	GRADED TRIAL #1	GRADED TRIAL #2	NOTES:
1. ◆	Identify the correct patient electronic health record where the error was made.				
2. ◆	Locate the error within the record.				
3. ★	Using the rules associated with the software you are using, make the appropriate correction within the medical record.				
4. ★	Sign off on the changes as necessary, according to the steps required within the software program.				
5. ◆	Verify the change made is correct before closing the patient's electronic health record.				

© 2015 Pearson Education, Inc.

Name: _____

Date: _____

Document: Enter the appropriate information in the chart below.

Grading

Points Earned	_____		
Points Possible	_____	36	36
Percent Grade (Points Earned/Points Possible)	_____		
PASS:	_____	❏ YES ❏ NO ❏ N/A	❏ YES ❏ NO ❏ N/A

Instructor Sign-Off

Instructor: _____ **Date:** _____

© 2015 Pearson Education, Inc.

Name: _____

Date: _____

Procedure 13-1:

Use Computer Software to Maintain Office Systems

Objective: Use computer software to maintain office systems correctly within the time limit set by the instructor.

Supplies: Computer with spreadsheet software, list of equipment to enter into the computer.

Affective Behaviors: Affective behaviors provide a professional approach to a skill that enhances the patient encounter. These behaviors may also display sensitivity to patients' rights, enhance communication, convey an understanding of laws and regulations, and/or provide an overall professional component to the medical assisting profession. Pay close attention to these skills, which appear in **_bold, italicized_** font.

Notes to the Student:

_____

_____

_____

_____

_____

_____

Skills Assessment Requirements

Read and familiarize yourself with the procedure; complete the minimum practice requirements (MPRs). Document each MPR using proper charting technique. Complete each procedure within a reasonable amount of time, with a minimum of 85 percent accuracy.

Name: _____

Date: _____

POINT VALUE ◆ = 3–6 points ★ = 7–9 points		PRACTICE TRIAL	GRADED TRIAL #1	GRADED TRIAL #2	NOTES:
1. ◆	Launch the spreadsheet software.				
2. ◆	Using the list of equipment, enter each piece of equipment onto a separate line on the spreadsheet.				
3. ◆	Enter the date each piece of equipment was purchased or leased by the medical office.				
4. ★	Enter the name of the manufacturer that supplied the piece of equipment.				
5. ◆	Enter the type of maintenance the piece of equipment needs on a regular basis.				
6. ◆	Enter information about the needed maintenance, such as the name of the company that performs the repairs, and the schedule for which the equipment must be maintained. ***Enter as much information as possible so as to maintain time efficiency at the time of repairs and maintenance.***				

© 2015 Pearson Education, Inc.

Name: _____

Date: _____

Document: Enter the appropriate information in the chart below.

Grading

Points Earned	_____		
Points Possible	_____	39	39
Percent Grade (Points Earned/Points Possible)	_____		
PASS:	_____	❏ YES ❏ NO ❏ N/A	❏ YES ❏ NO ❏ N/A

Instructor Sign-Off

Instructor: _____ **Date:** _____

© 2015 Pearson Education, Inc.

Name: _____

Date: _____

Procedure 13-2:

Use an Internet Search Engine

Objective: Use the computer to search for a topic via an Internet search engine correctly within the time limit set by the instructor.

Supplies: A computer with Internet access.

Notes to the Student:

_____

_____

_____

_____

_____

_____

Skills Assessment Requirements

Read and familiarize yourself with the procedure; complete the minimum practice requirements (MPRs). Document each MPR using proper charting technique. Complete each procedure within a reasonable amount of time, with a minimum of 85 percent accuracy.

Name: _____

Date: _____

POINT VALUE ◆ = 3–6 points ★ = 7–9 points		PRACTICE TRIAL	GRADED TRIAL #1	GRADED TRIAL #2	NOTES:
1. ◆	Turn on the computer.				
2. ◆	Launch an Internet browser.				
3. ◆	Visit the uniform resource locator (URL) of the search engine.				
4. ◆	Enter the search keywords.				
5. ◆	Visit retrieved Web sites to obtain the desired information.				
6. ◆	To refine the search, enter more or different key words.				

© 2015 Pearson Education, Inc.

Name: _____

Date: _____

Document: Enter the appropriate information in the chart below.

Grading

Points Earned	_____		
Points Possible	_____	36	36
Percent Grade (Points Earned/Points Possible)	_____		
PASS:	_____	❏ YES ❏ NO ❏ N/A	❏ YES ❏ NO ❏ N/A

Instructor Sign-Off

Instructor: _____ **Date:** _____

© 2015 Pearson Education, Inc.

Procedure 13-3:

Use the Computer to Verify Preferred Provider Status on an Insurance Company Web Site

Objective: Verify a provider's preferred status on an insurance company Web site within the time limit set by the instructor.

Supplies: Computer with Internet connection, insurance company's URL, name of target physician.

Notes to the Student:

_____

_____

_____

_____

_____

_____

_____

Skills Assessment Requirements

Read and familiarize yourself with the procedure; complete the minimum practice requirements (MPRs). Document each MPR using proper charting technique. Complete each procedure within a reasonable amount of time, with a minimum of 85 percent accuracy.

© 2015 Pearson Education, Inc.

Name: _____

Date: _____

POINT VALUE ◆ = 3–6 points ★ = 7–9 points	PRACTICE TRIAL	GRADED TRIAL #1	GRADED TRIAL #2	NOTES:
1. ◆ Using the computer, launch an Internet browser.				
2. ◆ Enter the URL of the insurance company.				
3. ◆ Navigate to the provider page or section.				
4. ◆ In the search field, enter the provider's name and/or location.				
5. ◆ Verify if the physician is preferred with the target insurance company.				

© 2015 Pearson Education, Inc.

Name: _____

Date: _____

Document: Enter the appropriate information in the chart below.

Grading

Points Earned	_____		
Points Possible	_____	30	30
Percent Grade (Points Earned/Points Possible)	_____		
PASS:	_____	❏ YES ❏ NO ❏ N/A	❏ YES ❏ NO ❏ N/A

Instructor Sign-Off

Instructor: _____ **Date:** _____

© 2015 Pearson Education, Inc.

Procedure 14-1:

Take Inventory of Administrative Equipment

Objective: Perform an inventory of administrative equipment correctly within the time limit set by the instructor.

Supplies: Paper, pen, computer with word-processing or spreadsheet software.

Affective Behaviors: Affective behaviors provide a professional approach to a skill that enhances the patient encounter. These behaviors may also display sensitivity to patients' rights, enhance communication, convey an understanding of laws and regulations, and/or provide an overall professional component to the medical assisting profession. Pay close attention to these skills, which appear in **bold, *italicized*** font.

Notes to the Student:

_____

_____

_____

_____

_____

_____

Skills Assessment Requirements

Read and familiarize yourself with the procedure; complete the minimum practice requirements (MPRs). Document each MPR using proper charting technique. Complete each procedure within a reasonable amount of time, with a minimum of 85 percent accuracy.

© 2015 Pearson Education, Inc.

POINT VALUE ◆ = 3–6 points ★ = 7–9 points		PRACTICE TRIAL	GRADED TRIAL #1	GRADED TRIAL #2	NOTES:
1. ◆	Locate all administrative equipment in the medical office.				
2. ★	List each piece of equipment with manufacturer name, serial number, and date of purchase, when known.				
3. ◆	Include information about the company maintaining the equipment.				
4. ◆	Include information about the supplies needed to maintain the equipment, including where those supplies are purchased.				
5. ◆	Using word-processing or spreadsheet software, create an inventory sheet of all equipment information. *The inventory sheet should be easy to read and should contain succinct information on all items, ensuring time efficacy.*				
6. ◆	Update the inventory sheet as needed when new equipment is purchased or older equipment is replaced.				

© 2015 Pearson Education, Inc.

Name: _____

Date: _____

Document: Enter the appropriate information in the chart below.

Grading

Points Earned	_____		
Points Possible	_____	39	39
Percent Grade (Points Earned/Points Possible)	_____		
PASS:	_____	❏ YES ❏ NO ❏ N/A	❏ YES ❏ NO ❏ N/A

Instructor Sign-Off

Instructor: _____   **Date:** _____

© 2015 Pearson Education, Inc.

Procedure 14-2:

Fax a Document

Objective: Fax a document using a fax machine correctly within the time limit set by the instructor.

Supplies: Document to be faxed, HIPAA-compliant fax cover sheet, pen, fax machine.

Affective Behaviors: Affective behaviors provide a professional approach to a skill that enhances the patient encounter. These behaviors may also display sensitivity to patients' rights, enhance communication, convey an understanding of laws and regulations, and/or provide an overall professional component to the medical assisting profession. Pay close attention to these skills, which appear in **bold, italicized** font.

Notes to the Student:

_____

_____

_____

_____

_____

_____

_____

Skills Assessment Requirements

Read and familiarize yourself with the procedure; complete the minimum practice requirements (MPRs). Document each MPR using proper charting technique. Complete each procedure within a reasonable amount of time, with a minimum of 85 percent accuracy.

© 2015 Pearson Education, Inc.

Name: _____

Date: _____

POINT VALUE ◆ = 3–6 points ★ = 7–9 points		PRACTICE TRIAL	GRADED TRIAL #1	GRADED TRIAL #2	NOTES:
1. ◆	Complete the **HIPAA-compliant fax cover sheet** with your own name, phone number, and clinic contact information.				
2. ◆	Fill in the name and fax number of the fax recipient.				
3. ◆	List the number of pages in the fax, including the cover sheet.				
4. ◆	Properly orient the fax cover sheet and document to be faxed in the fax machine.				
5. ◆	Dial the target fax number. **Prior to hitting the "send" button, double check that the fax number has been accurately entered.**				
6. ★	When the fax has been fully transmitted, remove the documents and file them with the fax confirmation sheet to the patient's file.				

© 2015 Pearson Education, Inc.

Name: _____

Date: _____

Document: Enter the appropriate information in the chart below.

Grading

Points Earned	_____		
Points Possible	_____	39	39
Percent Grade (Points Earned/Points Possible)	_____		
PASS:	_____	❏ YES ❏ NO ❏ N/A	❏ YES ❏ NO ❏ N/A

Instructor Sign-Off

Instructor: _____   **Date:** _____

© 2015 Pearson Education, Inc.

Procedure 14-3:

Perform Routine Maintenance of a Computer Printer

Objective: Perform routine maintenance of a computer printer correctly within the time limit set by the instructor.

Supplies: Paper, pen, computer printer, maintenance logbook.

Notes to the Student:

_____

_____

_____

_____

_____

Skills Assessment Requirements

Read and familiarize yourself with the procedure; complete the minimum practice requirements (MPRs). Document each MPR using proper charting technique. Complete each procedure within a reasonable amount of time, with a minimum of 85 percent accuracy.

© 2015 Pearson Education, Inc.

Name: _____

Date: _____

POINT VALUE ◆ = 3–6 points ★ = 7–9 points		PRACTICE TRIAL	GRADED TRIAL #1	GRADED TRIAL #2	NOTES:
1. ◆	Review the maintenance logbook for the computer printer.				
2. ◆	Following the manufacturer's directions, open the printer cover and remove the toner cartridge.				
3. ◆	Using the manufacturer-provided cleaning tool, clean any dust and spilled toner from within the printer.				
4. ◆	Replace the cleaning tool and the toner cartridge.				
5. ◆	Close the printer cover.				
6. ★	In the maintenance logbook, enter information about the maintenance, including the date and your signature.				

© 2015 Pearson Education, Inc.

Name: _____

Date: _____

Document: Enter the appropriate information in the chart below.

Grading

Points Earned	_____		
Points Possible	_____	39	39
Percent Grade (Points Earned/Points Possible)	_____		
PASS:	_____	❏ YES ❏ NO ❏ N/A	❏ YES ❏ NO ❏ N/A

Instructor Sign-Off

Instructor: _____ **Date:** _____

© 2015 Pearson Education, Inc.

Procedure 14-4:

Prepare a Purchase Order

Objective: Prepare a purchase order correctly within the time limit set by the instructor.

Supplies: List of needed supplies, purchase order form, pen, fax machine or telephone.

Notes to the Student:

_____

_____

_____

_____

_____

_____

_____

Skills Assessment Requirements

Read and familiarize yourself with the procedure; complete the minimum practice requirements (MPRs). Document each MPR using proper charting technique. Complete each procedure within a reasonable amount of time, with a minimum of 85 percent accuracy.

© 2015 Pearson Education, Inc.

Name: _____

Date: _____

POINT VALUE ◆ = 3–6 points ★ = 7–9 points		PRACTICE TRIAL	GRADED TRIAL #1	GRADED TRIAL #2	NOTES:
1. ◆	Review the list of needed supplies, grouping them according to the vendor they will be ordered from.				
2. ◆	Fill in the name and fax number of the company the supplies are to be ordered from.				
3. ★	List each supply individually on the purchase order, taking care to note the quantity needed and the part number associated with each item.				
4. ◆	If the physician's signature is required, obtain his or her signature. If it is not required, sign and date the form yourself.				
5. ★	If the purchase order can be faxed to the supplier, fax the document and make a note of the date and time the fax went through.				
6. ◆	If the purchase order cannot be faxed to the supplier, call the supplier and place the order over the telephone. Document the name of the person you spoke to and the date and time of the call.				
7. ◆	File the purchase order in a folder for pending orders.				

© 2015 Pearson Education, Inc.

Name: _____

Date: _____

Document: Enter the appropriate information in the chart below.

Grading

Points Earned	_____		
Points Possible	_____	48	48
Percent Grade (Points Earned/Points Possible)	_____		
PASS:	_____	❏ YES ❏ NO ❏ N/A	❏ YES ❏ NO ❏ N/A

Instructor Sign-Off

Instructor: _____ **Date:** _____

© 2015 Pearson Education, Inc.

Procedure 14-5:

Receive a Supply Shipment

Objective: Receive a supply shipment correctly within the time limit set by the instructor.

Supplies: Box of supplies, packing slip, supply inventory logbook, pen.

Notes to the Student:

_____

_____

_____

_____

_____

_____

Skills Assessment Requirements

Read and familiarize yourself with the procedure; complete the minimum practice requirements (MPRs). Document each MPR using proper charting technique. Complete each procedure within a reasonable amount of time, with a minimum of 85 percent accuracy.

© 2015 Pearson Education, Inc.

POINT VALUE ◆ = 3–6 points ★ = 7–9 points		PRACTICE TRIAL	GRADED TRIAL #1	GRADED TRIAL #2	NOTES:
1. ◆	Open the box of supplies and locate the packing slip.				
2. ◆	Remove each item from the box, checking it on the packing slip.				
3. ◆	On the packing slip, circle any missing supplies.				
4. ◆	Put the supplies away, newer ones behind older ones.				
5. ◆	Note in the supply log that the supplies have been received.				
6. ★	When any supplies on the packing slip are absent from the shipment, notify the supplier.				
7. ◆	When any supplies on the packing slip are on back-order, retain the slip until the backordered supplies arrive.				
8. ★	When the packing slip also serves as an invoice, route it to the accounts payable department.				
9. ◆	Discard packing materials appropriately.				

© 2015 Pearson Education, Inc.

Name: _____

Date: _____

Document: Enter the appropriate information in the chart below.

Grading

Points Earned	_____		
Points Possible	_____	60	60
Percent Grade (Points Earned/Points Possible)	_____		
PASS:	_____	❏ YES ❏ NO ❏ N/A	❏ YES ❏ NO ❏ N/A

Instructor Sign-Off

Instructor: _____ **Date:** _____

© 2015 Pearson Education, Inc.

Name: _____

Date: _____

Procedure 15-1:

Create an Office Brochure

Objective: Create an office brochure correctly within the time limit set by the instructor.

Supplies: Computer with word-processing and/or publishing software, list of information the physician would like in an office brochure.

Affective Behaviors: Affective behaviors provide a professional approach to a skill that enhances the patient encounter. These behaviors may also display sensitivity to patients' rights, enhance communication, convey an understanding of laws and regulations, and/or provide an overall professional component to the medical assisting profession. Pay close attention to these skills, which appear in **_bold, italicized_** font.

Notes to the Student:

_____

_____

_____

_____

_____

_____

_____

Skills Assessment Requirements

Read and familiarize yourself with the procedure; complete the minimum practice requirements (MPRs). Document each MPR using proper charting technique. Complete each procedure within a reasonable amount of time, with a minimum of 85 percent accuracy.

© 2015 Pearson Education, Inc.

Name: _____

Date: _____

POINT VALUE ◆ = 3–6 points ★ = 7–9 points		PRACTICE TRIAL	GRADED TRIAL #1	GRADED TRIAL #2	NOTES:
1. ◆	Gather information on the brochure's subject.				
2. ◆	Launch the word-processing and/or publishing software.				
3. ◆	Create a title for the brochure, such as "Living with Diabetes."				
4. ◆	**Add information to the brochure in an easy-to-read format. Use simple terms rather than medical terminology.**				
5. ◆	Add information regarding where the patient can look for further resources, such as Web sites.				
6. ◆	Include the office's name, address, and telephone number.				
7. ★	Check for typographical and grammatical errors.				
8. ★	Print the brochure, and **give it to the physician for review before making copies for patients.**				

© 2015 Pearson Education, Inc.

Name: _____

Date: _____

Document: Enter the appropriate information in the chart below.

Grading

Points Earned	_____		
Points Possible	_____	54	54
Percent Grade (Points Earned/Points Possible)	_____		
PASS:	_____	❏ YES ❏ NO ❏ N/A	❏ YES ❏ NO ❏ N/A

Instructor Sign-Off

Instructor: _____   **Date:** _____

Procedure 15-2:

Create a Procedure for the Procedure Manual

Objective: Create a procedure for the procedure manual correctly within the time limit set by the instructor.

Supplies: Computer with word-processing software.

Affective Behaviors: Affective behaviors provide a professional approach to a skill that enhances the patient encounter. These behaviors may also display sensitivity to patients' rights, enhance communication, convey an understanding of laws and regulations, and/or provide an overall professional component to the medical assisting profession. Pay close attention to these skills, which appear in **_bold, italicized_** font.

Notes to the Student:

_____

_____

_____

_____

_____

_____

_____

Skills Assessment Requirements

Read and familiarize yourself with the procedure; complete the minimum practice requirements (MPRs). Document each MPR using proper charting technique. Complete each procedure within a reasonable amount of time, with a minimum of 85 percent accuracy.

© 2015 Pearson Education, Inc.

POINT VALUE ◆ = 3–6 points ★ = 7–9 points		PRACTICE TRIAL	GRADED TRIAL #1	GRADED TRIAL #2	NOTES:
1. ◆	Determine the type of procedure to be created.				
2. ◆	Gather the information on how this procedure is to be performed.				
3. ◆	Title the procedure (e.g., "Policy: Sorting Incoming Mail"), and determine if it will be listed under administrative, clinical, infection control, personnel, or quality improvement and risk management.				
4. ◆	Describe the policy's purpose (e.g., "Purpose: To describe the method of routing incoming mail to appropriate staff").				
5. ◆	List each step in the procedure. **Ensure that each step fits well within the scope of practice and is succinct and time efficient.**				
6. ★	Print the procedure and give it to the office manager for approval.				
7. ◆	Once approved, place the procedure in the office procedure manual.				

© 2015 Pearson Education, Inc.

Name: _____

Date: _____

Document: Enter the appropriate information in the chart below.

Grading

Points Earned	_____		
Points Possible	_____	45	45
Percent Grade (Points Earned/Points Possible)	_____		
PASS:	_____	❏ YES ❏ NO ❏ N/A	❏ YES ❏ NO ❏ N/A

Instructor Sign-Off

Instructor: _____ **Date:** _____

© 2015 Pearson Education, Inc.

Name: _____

Date: _____

Procedure 16-1:

Maintain a List of Community Resources for Emergencies

Objective: To maintain a list of community resources for emergencies.

Supplies: Notepad and pen, computer with word-processing software, Internet connection with search engine availability, phonebook, printer, printer paper.

Notes to the Student:

_____

_____

_____

_____

_____

_____

Skills Assessment Requirements

Read and familiarize yourself with the procedure; complete the minimum practice requirements (MPRs). Document each MPR using proper charting technique. Complete each procedure within a reasonable amount of time, with a minimum of 85 percent accuracy.

© 2015 Pearson Education, Inc.

POINT VALUE ◆ = 3–6 points ★ = 7–9 points		PRACTICE TRIAL	GRADED TRIAL #1	GRADED TRIAL #2	NOTES:
1. ★	Using a notepad and pen, compile a list of community resources that are available either during or after an emergency. Some resources you will want to be sure to include are: • Poison Control Center • Local fire and police departments, main numbers not 9-1-1 • Local chapter of the Red Cross • Federal Emergency Management Agency (FEMA) • Local food banks • Local housing shelters • Emergency medical facilities, including hospitals and urgent care facilities • Other facilities that are unique to your area that can provide assistance during or after an emergency				
2. ◆	Using an Internet search engine or a local telephone book, write down the contact telephone numbers and corresponding Web sites for each company and organization listed.				
3. ◆	Open the word-processing software that is on the computer.				

© 2015 Pearson Education, Inc.

4. ◆	Create a new document that clearly and neatly organizes this information. You may want to choose to create a brochure with a description of each agency, or you may choose to create a single sheet of information that displays the information in a table format.				
5. ◆	After you have created the information in the Word document, review the information for accuracy.				
6. ◆	Using the software tools, perform a spelling and grammar check, making changes as necessary.				
7. ◆	Review the document for a second time to check for information accuracy, and perform a second spelling and grammar check.				
8. ◆	Save the document in the appropriate file on the computer.				
9. ★	Print the document and show it to the office manager or physician for approval.				
10. ◆	Once final approval is given, make multiple copies to have on hand to pass out to patients as necessary.				

© 2015 Pearson Education, Inc.

Document: Enter the appropriate information in the chart below.

Grading

Points Earned	_____		
Points Possible	_____	63	63
Percent Grade (Points Earned/Points Possible)	_____		
PASS:	_____	❏ YES ❏ NO ❏ N/A	❏ YES ❏ NO ❏ N/A

Instructor Sign-Off

Instructor: _____   **Date:** _____

© 2015 Pearson Education, Inc.

Name: _____

Date: _____

Procedure 16-2:

Perform Adult Rescue Breathing and One-Rescuer CPR

Objective: Using the supplies and equipment listed below, demonstrate how to administer rescue breathing for an adult and one-rescuer CPR for an adult.

Supplies: Approved mannequin, gloves, ventilator mask, mouth guard.

Affective Behaviors: Affective behaviors provide a professional approach to a skill that enhances the patient encounter. These behaviors may also display sensitivity to patients' rights, enhance communication, convey an understanding of laws and regulations, and/or provide an overall professional component to the medical assisting profession. Pay close attention to these skills, which appear in **bold, *italicized*** font.

Notes to the Student:

_____

_____

_____

_____

_____

_____

_____

Skills Assessment Requirements

Read and familiarize yourself with the procedure; complete the minimum practice requirements (MPRs). Document each MPR using proper charting technique. Complete each procedure within a reasonable amount of time, with a minimum of 85 percent accuracy.

© 2015 Pearson Education, Inc.

Name: _____

Date: _____

POINT VALUE ◆ = 3–6 points ★ = 7–9 points		PRACTICE TRIAL	GRADED TRIAL #1	GRADED TRIAL #2	NOTES:
1. ◆	Assess the victim and determine if help is needed. Shout "Are you OK?" while gently shaking the victim's shoulders. **State your name and inform the victim that you are there to help.**				
2. ◆	If gloves are available, put them on. If you have a ventilator mask, place it on the victim.				
3. ◆	If the adult victim is determined to be unresponsive, activate EMS immediately by having someone else call 9-1-1 and retrieve an AED if available. If you are alone, begin the rescue sequence for 1 minute and then attempt to call 9-1-1 yourself. **Remain calm and collected during the next steps.**				
4. ★	Check the carotid artery for a pulse and assess for breathing, taking no more than 10 seconds.				
5. ★	If pulse is absent, position yourself and prepare for chest compressions: Kneel at the victim's side. Find the sternum and place the heel of one hand just below the nipple line. Place your other hand on top of the first hand, making sure to lift your fingers off the chest, using only the heels of your hands to administer compressions.				

© 2015 Pearson Education, Inc.

6. ★	Using the full weight of your upper body, perform 30 compressions at a depth of at least 2 inches in 18 seconds or less.				
7. ★	Put on a mouth guard, perform the head tilt–chin lift, and administer two rescue breaths. If your breaths do not cause the chest to rise, look in the victim's mouth and remove any object you see. If no object is seen, make a second attempt to administer a rescue breath. If the breath still does not enter the chest, proceed to abdominal thrusts for unconscious victims.				
8. ★	Continue with chest compressions and rescue breaths at a 30:2 ratio. After five complete cycles, reassess the patient by checking for breathing and a pulse at the carotid artery. To check for breathing, remove the mask, and place your ear near the patient's mouth to see if you can hear or feel breath, while at the same time observing the chest for rising and falling associated with breathing.				
9. ★	If a pulse is present, continue with rescue breaths at a rate of 1 every 5–8 seconds, or about 10–12 per minute. After 1 minute of rescue breathing, reassess the patient for breathing and pulse.				
10. ★	If neither is present, continue with compressions and rescue breaths at a 30:2 ratio until an AED is made available or until emergency medical services arrive and you are relieved from performing CPR.				

Name: _____

Date: _____

Document: Enter the appropriate information in the chart below.

Grading

Points Earned	_____		
Points Possible	_____	81	81
Percent Grade (Points Earned/Points Possible)	_____		
PASS:	_____	❏ YES ❏ NO ❏ N/A	❏ YES ❏ NO ❏ N/A

Instructor Sign-Off

Instructor: _____ **Date:** _____

© 2015 Pearson Education, Inc.

Name: _____

Date: _____

Procedure 16-3:

Respond to a Patient Who Has Fainted

Objective: Care correctly for a patient who has fainted within the time limit set by the instructor.

Supplies: Blanket, washcloths, footstool or box.

Affective Behaviors: Affective behaviors provide a professional approach to a skill that enhances the patient encounter. These behaviors may also display sensitivity to patients' rights, enhance communication, convey an understanding of laws and regulations, and/or provide an overall professional component to the medical assisting profession. Pay close attention to these skills, which appear in **bold, italicized** font.

Notes to the Student:

_____

_____

_____

_____

_____

_____

_____

Skills Assessment Requirements

Read and familiarize yourself with the procedure; complete the minimum practice requirements (MPRs). Document each MPR using proper charting technique. Complete each procedure within a reasonable amount of time, with a minimum of 85 percent accuracy.

© 2015 Pearson Education, Inc.

Name: _____

Date: _____

POINT VALUE ◆ = 3–6 points ★ = 7–9 points		PRACTICE TRIAL	GRADED TRIAL #1	GRADED TRIAL #2	NOTES:
1. ◆	If the patient says he is feeling faint, help him sit, bend forward, and place his head on his knees. If the patient collapses with no warning, do not move him. He might have sustained a neck or back injury.				
2. ◆	**Remain calm, notify the physician immediately, and always act within your scope of practice.**				
3. ◆	Loosen any tight clothing, and cover the patient with the blanket for warmth. If the patient has fainted due to heat exhaustion, place cold washcloths on the patient's neck and wrists.				
4. ◆	If the physician directs, use the footstool to support the patient's legs in a raised position.				
5. ◆	If the physician directs, call for emergency services.				
6. ★	Once the emergency passes, document all activities in the patient's medical record.				

© 2015 Pearson Education, Inc.

Name: _____

Date: _____

Document: Enter the appropriate information in the chart below.

Grading

Points Earned	_____		
Points Possible	_____	39	39
Percent Grade (Points Earned/Points Possible)	_____		
PASS:	_____	❏ YES ❏ NO ❏ N/A	❏ YES ❏ NO ❏ N/A

Instructor Sign-Off

Instructor: _____ **Date:** _____

© 2015 Pearson Education, Inc.

Procedure 16-4:

Administer Oxygen to a Patient

Objective: Using the supplies and equipment listed below, demonstrate how to administer oxygen therapy to an adult.

Supplies: Portable oxygen tank, pressure regulator, flow meter, nasal cannula with connecting tubing, oxygen mask with connecting tubing.

Notes to the Student:

_____

_____

_____

_____

_____

_____

Skills Assessment Requirements

Read and familiarize yourself with the procedure; complete the minimum practice requirements (MPRs). Document each MPR using proper charting technique. Complete each procedure within a reasonable amount of time, with a minimum of 85 percent accuracy.

© 2015 Pearson Education, Inc.

Name: _____

Date: _____

POINT VALUE ◆ = 3–6 points ★ = 7–9 points		PRACTICE TRIAL	GRADED TRIAL #1	GRADED TRIAL #2	NOTES:
1. ◆	Gather all equipment.				
2. ◆	Wash your hands.				
3. ★	Identify the patient and explain what you are about to do.				
4. ◆	Check the pressure gauge on the oxygen tank to verify the amount of oxygen in the tank.				
5. ◆	Open the cylinder on the oxygen tank one full counterclockwise turn and attach the connective tubing to the flow meter.				
6. ◆	Attach either the nasal cannula or the oxygen mask to the connective tubing.				
7. ◆	When using a nasal cannula, insert the cannula tips into the patient's nostrils and loop the tubing behind the patient's ears.				
8. ◆	When using an oxygen mask, place the oxygen mask over the patient's nose and mouth and slip the elastic cord over his or her head. Adjust the cord so that the mask fits tightly yet comfortably on the patient's face.				
9. ◆	Adjust the administration of the oxygen to the flow ordered by the physician.				
10. ◆	Verify that oxygen is flowing through the nasal cannula or oxygen mask.				

© 2015 Pearson Education, Inc.

11. ◆	Wash your hands.				
12. ◆	Document the procedure, including the flow rate of oxygen being given to the patient and the method of delivery (nasal cannula or oxygen mask).				

© 2015 Pearson Education, Inc.

Document: Enter the appropriate information in the chart below.

Grading

Points Earned	_____		
Points Possible	_____	75	75
Percent Grade (Points Earned/Points Possible)	_____		
PASS:	_____	❏ YES ❏ NO ❏ N/A	❏ YES ❏ NO ❏ N/A

Instructor Sign-Off

Instructor: _____ **Date:** _____

© 2015 Pearson Education, Inc.

Procedure 16-5:

Use an Automated External Defibrillator (AED)

Objective: Using the supplies and equipment listed below, demonstrate how to use an AED.

Supplies: Practice AED machine, patient chart, mannequin.

Affective Behaviors: Affective behaviors provide a professional approach to a skill that enhances the patient encounter. These behaviors may also display sensitivity to patients' rights, enhance communication, convey an understanding of laws and regulations, and/or provide an overall professional component to the medical assisting profession. Pay close attention to these skills, which appear in **bold, italicized** font.

Notes to the Student:

_____

_____

_____

_____

_____

_____

_____

Skills Assessment Requirements

Read and familiarize yourself with the procedure; complete the minimum practice requirements (MPRs). Document each MPR using proper charting technique. Complete each procedure within a reasonable amount of time, with a minimum of 85 percent accuracy.

© 2015 Pearson Education, Inc.

Name: _____

Date: _____

POINT VALUE ◆ = 3–6 points ★ = 7–9 points		PRACTICE TRIAL	GRADED TRIAL #1	GRADED TRIAL #2	NOTES:
1. ◆	**State your name and inform the victim that you are there to help.** Place the AED next to the victim's left ear. This position allows the rescuers clear access to the chest and airway for continued rescue measures.				
2. ★	Turn the AED on and follow the voice prompts. **Remain calm and collected during the next steps.**				
3. ◆	You will be prompted to attach the electrode pads to the patient's chest, on the sternum and at the apex of the heart, following the diagram for correct placement.				
4. ◆	Next, you will be directed to allow the machine to analyze the heart rhythm to determine if it is a shockable rhythm. CPR should cease while the machine is analyzing.				
5. ◆	The machine will begin a charging sequence prior to shocking and will warn rescuers to stand back. The voice prompt will then tell you to press the "shock" button to administer the electrical current to the patient.				
6. ★	If the machine indicates "No shock is advised," assess the patient for breathing and circulation. Continue CPR as needed until advanced medical personnel arrive. **Always act within your scope of practice.**				

© 2015 Pearson Education, Inc.

Name: _____

Date: _____

Document: Enter the appropriate information in the chart below.

Grading

Points Earned	_____		
Points Possible	_____	81	81
Percent Grade (Points Earned/Points Possible)	_____		
PASS:	_____	❏ YES ❏ NO ❏ N/A	❏ YES ❏ NO ❏ N/A

Instructor Sign-Off

Instructor: _____ **Date:** _____

© 2015 Pearson Education, Inc.

Procedure 16-6:

Respond to an Adult with an Airway Obstruction

Objective: Using the supplies and equipment listed below, demonstrate how to administer the Heimlich maneuver to an adult.

Supplies: Approved mannequin, gloves, ventilation mask with one-way valve for an unconscious victim.

Notes to the Student:

_____

_____

_____

_____

_____

_____

Skills Assessment Requirements

Read and familiarize yourself with the procedure; complete the minimum practice requirements (MPRs). Document each MPR using proper charting technique. Complete each procedure within a reasonable amount of time, with a minimum of 85 percent accuracy.

Name: _____

Date: _____

POINT VALUE ◆ = 3–6 points ★ = 7–9 points		PRACTICE TRIAL	GRADED TRIAL #1	GRADED TRIAL #2	NOTES:
1. ★	Establish that the victim is choking by asking, "Are you choking?" or "Can you speak?" If the victim indicates she is choking by a head shake or the universal choking sign, tell her you are going to begin emergency treatment and direct someone to call 9-1-1.				
2. ◆	Stand behind the victim with your feet slightly apart, placing one foot between the victim's feet and one to the outside. This stance will give you greater stability, and if the victim should pass out, you can safely guide the patient to the ground by sliding him or her down your thigh.				
3. ◆	Place the index finger of one hand at the person's navel or belt buckle. If the victim is a pregnant woman, place your finger above the enlarged uterus.				
4. ◆	Make a fist with your other hand and place it, thumb side to victim, above your other hand. If the person is very pregnant, the uterus is pushing the stomach and other internal organs under the rib cage, and you may have to do chest compressions.				
5. ◆	Place your marking hand over your curled fist and begin to give quick inward and upward thrusts.				

© 2015 Pearson Education, Inc.

6. ◆	There is no set number of thrusts to give to an adult who remains conscious. Continue to give thrusts until the object is removed or the victim becomes unconscious.				
7. ◆	If the victim becomes unconscious, gently lower him or her to the ground.				
8. ◆	Activate EMS and put on gloves.				
9. ★	Immediately begin CPR with 30 chest compressions and two rescue breaths.				
10. ★	Before administering rescue breaths, open the airway with the head tilt–chin lift, and look for a foreign body in the victim's mouth, and remove if visible. Blind finger sweeps are no longer recommended and should not be performed.				
11. ◆	Continue with cycles of 30 compressions and two rescue breaths until the foreign body is expelled or advance medical personnel arrive to relieve you.				

© 2015 Pearson Education, Inc.

Name: _____

Date: _____

Document: Enter the appropriate information in the chart below.

Grading

Points Earned	_____		
Points Possible	_____	75	75
Percent Grade (Points Earned/Points Possible)	_____		
PASS:	_____	❏ YES ❏ NO ❏ N/A	❏ YES ❏ NO ❏ N/A

Instructor Sign-Off

Instructor: _____ Date: _____

© 2015 Pearson Education, Inc.

Procedure 16-7:

Remove an Airway Obstruction in an Infant

Objective: Remove an airway obstruction from an infant correctly within the time limit set by the instructor.

Supplies: Disposable gloves, infant mannequin.

Affective Behaviors: Affective behaviors provide a professional approach to a skill that enhances the patient encounter. These behaviors may also display sensitivity to patients' rights, enhance communication, convey an understanding of laws and regulations, and/or provide an overall professional component to the medical assisting profession. Pay close attention to these skills, which appear in **bold, italicized** font.

Notes to the Student:

_____

_____

_____

_____

_____

_____

Skills Assessment Requirements

Read and familiarize yourself with the procedure; complete the minimum practice requirements (MPRs). Document each MPR using proper charting technique. Complete each procedure within a reasonable amount of time, with a minimum of 85 percent accuracy.

© 2015 Pearson Education, Inc.

Name: _____

Date: _____

POINT VALUE ◆ = 3–6 points ★ = 7–9 points	PRACTICE TRIAL	GRADED TRIAL #1	GRADED TRIAL #2	NOTES:
1. ◆ Call for a coworker to dial 9-1-1 for emergency services. *Inform the patient's parent or guardian of your name and that you are going to help. Remain calm to calm those around you.*				
2. ★ Open the infant's mouth and look to see if an object is visible. If so, use your finger to sweep the object from the infant's mouth. If the object is NOT visible, do not blindly sweep your finger through the infant's mouth as you may push the object further back into the throat.				
3. ◆ Place the baby face down over your forearm and across your thigh. The infant's head should be lower than the trunk, and you should support the infant's head and neck with one hand.				
4. ◆ Using the heel of your free hand, administer five blows to the infant's back between the shoulder blades.				
5. ◆ Turn the infant over, keeping the head lower than the trunk, and administer five thrusts to the midsternal area of the infant.				

© 2015 Pearson Education, Inc.

6. ★	Look into the infant's mouth to see if the object is visible. If so, sweep your finger through the mouth to remove the object. If not, administer two rescue breaths into the infant by covering the infant's nose and mouth completely with your own mouth.				
7. ◆	Repeat the above sequence until the object is dislodged or help arrives.				
8. ★	Once the emergency passes, document all activities in the patient's medical record.				

Document: Enter the appropriate information in the chart below.

Grading

Points Earned	_____		
Points Possible	_____	57	57
Percent Grade (Points Earned/Points Possible)	_____		
PASS:	_____	❏ YES ❏ NO ❏ N/A	❏ YES ❏ NO ❏ N/A

Instructor Sign-Off

Instructor: _____   **Date:** _____

© 2015 Pearson Education, Inc.

Procedure 16-8:

Control Bleeding

Objective: Control bleeding in a patient correctly within the time limit set by the instructor.

Supplies: Disposable gloves, personal protective equipment (gown, eye protection, mask), sterile dressing, bandage, biohazard waste container.

Affective Behaviors: Affective behaviors provide a professional approach to a skill that enhances the patient encounter. These behaviors may also display sensitivity to patients' rights, enhance communication, convey an understanding of laws and regulations, and/or provide an overall professional component to the medical assisting profession. Pay close attention to these skills, which appear in **bold, italicized** font.

Notes to the Student:

_____

_____

_____

_____

_____

_____

Skills Assessment Requirements

Read and familiarize yourself with the procedure; complete the minimum practice requirements (MPRs). Document each MPR using proper charting technique. Complete each procedure within a reasonable amount of time, with a minimum of 85 percent accuracy.

© 2015 Pearson Education, Inc.

Name: _____

Date: _____

POINT VALUE ◆ = 3–6 points ★ = 7–9 points		PRACTICE TRIAL	GRADED TRIAL #1	GRADED TRIAL #2	NOTES:
1. ★	Notify a coworker to alert the physician. If a physician is not available in the office, notify the coworker to alert emergency personnel. **Always act within your scope of practice.**				
2. ◆	Assemble the necessary equipment and supplies. **Remain calm and try to calm those around you.**				
3. ◆	Wash your hands.				
4. ◆	Don the personal protective equipment.				
5. ◆	Open the sterile dressings, apply several layers directly to the wound, and apply direct pressure.				
6. ◆	Wrap the wound with bandage. If the wound continues to bleed, apply more sterile dressing and bandaging material. Continue to apply direct pressure.				
7. ◆	If the wound continues to bleed, and if it is located on an extremity, raise the extremity to a level above the patient's heart.				
8. ◆	If the bleeding continues, apply pressure to the appropriate artery.				
9. ◆	Once the bleeding is under control, dispose of all contaminated materials in the biohazard waste container.				
10. ◆	Wash your hands.				
11. ★	Once the emergency passes, document all activities in the patient's medical record.				

© 2015 Pearson Education, Inc.

Name: _____

Date: _____

Document: Enter the appropriate information in the chart below.

Grading

Points Earned	_____		
Points Possible	_____	72	72
Percent Grade (Points Earned/Points Possible)	_____		
PASS:	_____	❏ YES ❏ NO ❏ N/A	❏ YES ❏ NO ❏ N/A

Instructor Sign-Off

Instructor: _____ **Date:** _____

Procedure 16-9:

Develop a Safety Plan for Employees and Patients: Fire Evacuation

Objective: To develop a safety plan for employees and patients in the event fire evacuation is necessary.

Supplies: Pen, paper, computer with word-processing software, printer, copy machine, diagram of building evacuation routes.

Notes to the Student:

_____

_____

_____

_____

_____

_____

_____

Skills Assessment Requirements

Read and familiarize yourself with the procedure; complete the minimum practice requirements (MPRs). Document each MPR using proper charting technique. Complete each procedure within a reasonable amount of time, with a minimum of 85 percent accuracy.

© 2015 Pearson Education, Inc.

Name: _____

Date: _____

POINT VALUE ◆ = 3–6 points ★ = 7–9 points		PRACTICE TRIAL	GRADED TRIAL #1	GRADED TRIAL #2	NOTES:
1. ◆	Using word-processing software, create a new document that will outline the components of the safety plan.				
2. ◆	Clearly identify the evacuation routes to emergency exits for every room within the building. Include copies of the evacuation routes with the final and completed safety plan. If evacuation routes do not exist, they must be created.				
3. ◆	In the document, identify the safety zones, outside of the office building, where everyone will gather after evacuation. If possible, include photos of the safety zone or maps of the outside area clearly indicating the zone.				
4. ◆	Create a delineation chart that outlines responsibilities of office staff members in the event of a fire. The following tasks will require an assignment of responsibility: **a.** Activate fire rescue and emergency medical services by dialing 9-1-1. **b.** Close doors and windows (if safe to do so). **c.** Secure and remove the first aid kit upon exiting the office during evacuation (only if safe to do so).				

© 2015 Pearson Education, Inc.

5. ◆	In the document, create a section that specifically pertains to patient safety. Include the following information: **a.** Identify which office staff member will be in charge of directing and assisting the patients during evacuation. Remind patients that elevators may not be used in the event of a fire. **b.** Identify which office staff members will be in charge of checking that reception area and patient bathrooms have been evacuated. **c.** Identify which staff member will be in charge of retrieving the emergency first aid kit and transporting it to the safety zone, in the event that minor injuries are sustained during evacuation. **d.** Identify the office physician who will be responsible for evaluating and treating patients at the safety zone prior to the arrival of emergency personnel.				
6. ◆	In the document, create a section that specifically pertains to employee safety. Include the following information: **a.** Identify which office staff member will be in charge of checking that employee bathrooms, break room, laboratory, and other employee-only areas have been evacuated. **b.** Identify which office staff member will be in charge of taking a roll call at the safety zone to ensure that all office personnel have evacuated the building.				

7. ◆	The fire safety plan should also include the following information: **a.** When smoke alarm batteries should be replaced. **b.** When maintenance checks on fire extinguishers should occur. **c.** Ensuring that emergency first aid kits are fully stocked with products within expiration dates. **d.** Contact information for the insurance company that insures the medical office building.				
8. ◆	Perform grammar and spell-check within the document, and save the file.				
9. ◆	Print the document for review by the office manager and/or office physicians. Once approved, place a copy in the medical office's policy and procedure folder.				
10. ◆	Make copies of the fire safety plan and distribute it to all employees for review and discussion.				
11. ◆	Train all office staff on the fire safety plan within the first 10 days of hire.				

© 2015 Pearson Education, Inc.

Name: _____

Date: _____

Document: Enter the appropriate information in the chart below.

Grading

Points Earned	_____		
Points Possible	_____	66	66
Percent Grade (Points Earned/Points Possible)	_____		
PASS:	_____	❏ YES ❏ NO ❏ N/A	❏ YES ❏ NO ❏ N/A

Instructor Sign-Off

Instructor: _____ **Date:** _____

© 2015 Pearson Education, Inc.

Name: _____

Date: _____

Procedure 16-10:

Develop an Environmental Safety Plan

Objective: Develop an environmental safety plan with correct items in the time designated by the instructor.

Supplies: Pen, paper, computer, copy machine, various emergency supplies, waterproof containers.

Affective Behaviors: Affective behaviors provide a professional approach to a skill that enhances the patient encounter. These behaviors may also display sensitivity to patients' rights, enhance communication, convey an understanding of laws and regulations, and/or provide an overall professional component to the medical assisting profession. Pay close attention to these skills, which appear in **bold, *italicized*** font.

Notes to the Student:

_____

_____

_____

_____

_____

_____

Skills Assessment Requirements

Read and familiarize yourself with the procedure; complete the minimum practice requirements (MPRs). Document each MPR using proper charting technique. Complete each procedure within a reasonable amount of time, with a minimum of 85 percent accuracy.

© 2015 Pearson Education, Inc.

Name: _____

Date: _____

POINT VALUE ◆ = 3–6 points ★ = 7–9 points		PRACTICE TRIAL	GRADED TRIAL #1	GRADED TRIAL #2	NOTES:
1. ★	Create an emergency kit that can be used by your office in the event of an environmental emergency. Supplies may include: • Flashlights • Batteries • Bottles of water • Nonperishable food • Bandages • Alcohol and hydrogen peroxide • Blankets • Vinyl or latex gloves • Tweezers, scissors • Medication—ibuprofen, acetaminophen, antihistamines, antibiotic ointment, tetanus vaccines, etc. • Battery-powered radio				
2. ◆	Enclose the kit in a waterproof container.				
3. ◆	Place the kit in a safe area, such as a medicine closet or storage closet.				
4. ★	Create evacuation plans and make sure that every room in the medical office shows a detailed exit route. **Proper planning will reduce the stress level during the time of an emergency.**				
5. ★	Create a delineation chart that outlines responsibilities of office staff members in the event of an emergency. **Prior to creating the chart, ask your fellow staff if there are certain responsibilities they might prefer.**				

© 2015 Pearson Education, Inc.

6. ◆	Create a list of "safety zones" that can be used in the event of an emergency. For instance: • A safety zone in the event of a tornado. • A safety zone in the event of a flood. **_Once again, planning ahead may reduce stress levels during an actual emergency._**				
7. ◆	Make photocopies of the safety zone list, evacuation plan, and delineation chart for everyone in the office. **_Laminate and hang copies in the employee break room._**				
8. ★	**_Train all office staff on the environmental exposure plan within 10 days of hire._**				

© 2015 Pearson Education, Inc.

Name: _____

Date: _____

Document: Enter the appropriate information in the chart below.

Grading

Points Earned	_____		
Points Possible	_____	60	60
Percent Grade (Points Earned/Points Possible)	_____		
PASS:	_____	❏ YES ❏ NO ❏ N/A	❏ YES ❏ NO ❏ N/A

Instructor Sign-Off

Instructor: _____ **Date:** _____

© 2015 Pearson Education, Inc.

Name: _____

Date: _____

Procedure 16-11:

Participate in a Mock-Environmental Exposure: Responding to an Earthquake

Objective: To participate in a mock-environmental exposure by utilizing critical thinking skills and maintaining composure.

Supplies: Pen, paper.

Notes to the Student:

_____

_____

_____

_____

_____

_____

Skills Assessment Requirements

Read and familiarize yourself with the procedure; complete the minimum practice requirements (MPRs). Document each MPR using proper charting technique. Complete each procedure within a reasonable amount of time, with a minimum of 85 percent accuracy.

POINT VALUE ◆ = 3–6 points ★ = 7–9 points	PRACTICE TRIAL	GRADED TRIAL #1	GRADED TRIAL #2	NOTES:
1. ★ Evacuate the medical office or building as soon as safely possible. **a.** Make sure that staff members are following their given responsibilities during times of emergency. Someone (or a couple of staff members) must ensure the reception area, examination rooms, laboratory, physician offices, and bathrooms have all been evacuated of patients and staff members.				
2. ★ If it is reasonable and safe, gather the emergency supply kit on the way out of the building. **a.** Safety should always be your first priority. If the structure is unsafe, do not bother with anything other than evacuation and finding safety.				
3. ★ After evacuation, immediately go to the predetermined safety zone. **a.** As you, the medical assistant, are exiting the building, help patients and others by providing a calm voice of reassurance. Direct patients and their family members to congregate at the specified safety zone.				
4. ★ Provide assistance to the physicians as they begin to evaluate and treat injuries.				

© 2015 Pearson Education, Inc.

5. ★	Call 9-1-1 if there are injuries that are life threatening, serious, or unable to be treated at the scene.				
6. ★	Maintain your composure and continue to provide reassurance to those around you, addressing the needs and concerns of patients, coworkers, and physicians alike.				

© 2015 Pearson Education, Inc.

Document: Enter the appropriate information in the chart below.

Grading

Points Earned	_____		
Points Possible	_____	54	54
Percent Grade (Points Earned/Points Possible)	_____		
PASS:	_____	❏ YES ❏ NO ❏ N/A	❏ YES ❏ NO ❏ N/A

Instructor Sign-Off

Instructor: _____ **Date:** _____

© 2015 Pearson Education, Inc.

Procedure 17-1:

Calculate Deductible, Coinsurance, and Allowable Amounts

Objective: Calculate deductible, coinsurance, and allowable amounts correctly within the time limit set by the instructor.

Supplies: Pen, paper, insurance verification-of-benefits form, patient's insurance identification card, Explanation of Benefits (EOB) form, calculator.

Affective Behaviors: Affective behaviors provide a professional approach to a skill that enhances the patient encounter. These behaviors may also display sensitivity to patients' rights, enhance communication, convey an understanding of laws and regulations, and/or provide an overall professional component to the medical assisting profession. Pay close attention to these skills, which appear in **bold, italicized** font.

Notes to the Student:

_____

_____

_____

_____

_____

_____

_____

Skills Assessment Requirements

Read and familiarize yourself with the procedure; complete the minimum practice requirements (MPRs). Document each MPR using proper charting technique. Complete each procedure within a reasonable amount of time, with a minimum of 85 percent accuracy.

© 2015 Pearson Education, Inc.

Name: _____

Date: _____

POINT VALUE ◆ = 3–6 points ★ = 7–9 points		PRACTICE TRIAL	GRADED TRIAL #1	GRADED TRIAL #2	NOTES:
1. ◆	After the patient's insurance coverage has been verified, locate the information on the verification form regarding any deductible and coinsurance amount.				
2. ◆	*Inform the patient of the deductible amount that needs to be paid after the beginning of the calendar or fiscal year, before insurance payments become effective.*				
3. ◆	*Explain to the patient that the amount charged for any particular procedure in the medical office will likely be reduced to a lower amount (called the allowed amount) when processed by the insurance carrier.*				
4. ★	After the insurance payment is received, use the EOB form to identify the amount the insurance carrier allowed on the claim.				
5. ◆	Calculate the total allowed charges by adding together the allowed amount for each service.				
6. ◆	Subtract the deductible from the total of the allowed charges.				
7. ◆	Multiply the remaining allowed amount by the coinsurance percentage to determine the patient's coinsurance amount.				

© 2015 Pearson Education, Inc.

8. ★	Add the deductible to the coinsurance amount to determine the amount the patient needs to pay out of pocket for the visit.				
9. ★	**Explain the figures to the patient and collect the fees.**				

Name: _____

Date: _____

Document: Enter the appropriate information in the chart below.

Grading

Points Earned	_____		
Points Possible	_____	63	63
Percent Grade (Points Earned/Points Possible)	_____		
PASS:	_____	❑ YES ❑ NO ❑ N/A	❑ YES ❑ NO ❑ N/A

Instructor Sign-Off

Instructor: _____ **Date:** _____

© 2015 Pearson Education, Inc.

Name: _____

Date: _____

Procedure 17-2:

Verify a Patient's Insurance Eligibility

Objective: Verify a patient's insurance eligibility correctly within the time limit set by the instructor.

Supplies: Insurance identification card, patient's registration form, insurance verification of benefits worksheet, telephone or computer, paper, pen.

Affective Behaviors: Affective behaviors provide a professional approach to a skill that enhances the patient encounter. These behaviors may also display sensitivity to patients' rights, enhance communication, convey an understanding of laws and regulations, and/or provide an overall professional component to the medical assisting profession. Pay close attention to these skills, which appear in **bold, *italicized*** font.

Notes to the Student:

_____

_____

_____

_____

_____

_____

Skills Assessment Requirements

Read and familiarize yourself with the procedure; complete the minimum practice requirements (MPRs). Document each MPR using proper charting technique. Complete each procedure within a reasonable amount of time, with a minimum of 85 percent accuracy.

POINT VALUE ◆ = 3–6 points ★ = 7–9 points		PRACTICE TRIAL	GRADED TRIAL #1	GRADED TRIAL #2	NOTES:
1. ◆	Look at the patient's registration form and locate the patient's birthdate and the patient's relationship to the insured.				
2. ◆	Look at the patient's insurance identification card and locate the name of the insured, the insured's member identification number, and the telephone number of the insurance company.				
3. ◆	Call the insurance company at the provider customer service telephone number listed on the insurance identification card or access the insurance company's secure Web site, if available.				
4. ★	**When the customer service representative answers the call, write down the name of the customer service representative, and the date and time of the call.**				
5. ◆	Verify spelling of policyholder's name and birthdate.				
6. ◆	Verify patient's name and birthdate.				
7. ★	Verify coverage for type of service to be rendered, including frequency or number of visits.				
8. ◆	Verify when preauthorization is needed.				
9. ★	Verify patient's financial responsibility for deductible, copayment, or coinsurance amounts.				

© 2015 Pearson Education, Inc.

10. ★	Verify coordination of benefits rules if more than one policy covers the patient.				
11. ◆	Verify provider's participating or nonparticipating status.				
12. ◆	Verify the address where insurance claims are to be mailed or the payer number needed for electronic billing.				

© 2015 Pearson Education, Inc.

Document: Enter the appropriate information in the chart below.

Grading

Points Earned	_____		
Points Possible	_____	84	84
Percent Grade (Points Earned/Points Possible)	_____		
PASS:	_____	❏ YES ❏ NO ❏ N/A	❏ YES ❏ NO ❏ N/A

Instructor Sign-Off

Instructor: _____ **Date:** _____

© 2015 Pearson Education, Inc.

Name: _____

Date: _____

Procedure 17-3:

Obtain a Managed Care Referral

Objective: Obtain a managed care referral for a patient correctly within the time limit set by the instructor.

Supplies: Telephone, patient's medical chart, name and telephone number of patient's primary care provider.

Affective Behaviors: Affective behaviors provide a professional approach to a skill that enhances the patient encounter. These behaviors may also display sensitivity to patients' rights, enhance communication, convey an understanding of laws and regulations, and/or provide an overall professional component to the medical assisting profession. Pay close attention to these skills, which appear in **bold, _italicized_** font.

Notes to the Student:

_____

_____

_____

_____

_____

_____

Skills Assessment Requirements

Read and familiarize yourself with the procedure; complete the minimum practice requirements (MPRs). Document each MPR using proper charting technique. Complete each procedure within a reasonable amount of time, with a minimum of 85 percent accuracy.

© 2015 Pearson Education, Inc.

Name: _____

Date: _____

POINT VALUE ◆ = 3–6 points ★ = 7–9 points		PRACTICE TRIAL	GRADED TRIAL #1	GRADED TRIAL #2	NOTES:
1. ◆	Call the patient's primary care provider's office and ask for the person in charge of referrals.				
2. ◆	***Warmly greet the representative, state your name, and give the referral assistant the patient's information, including name and birthdate.***				
3. ◆	Inform the referral assistant of the need for a referral to the physician, including the reason for the patient's visit in the medical office.				
4. ◆	Ask the referral assistant if any information from the patient's file is needed to process the referral.				
5. ◆	Ask the referral assistant when to expect the referral. If needed, provide the office fax number for information transmittal. ***Thank the referral assistant for his or her guidance and bid the assistant a good day.***				
6. ★	Document in the patient's file the content of the telephone call.				
7. ◆	Notify the physician and the patient of the content of the telephone call.				

© 2015 Pearson Education, Inc.

Name: _____

Date: _____

Document: Enter the appropriate information in the chart below.

Grading

Points Earned	_____		
Points Possible	_____	45	45
Percent Grade (Points Earned/Points Possible)	_____		
PASS:	_____	❏ YES ❏ NO ❏ N/A	❏ YES ❏ NO ❏ N/A

Instructor Sign-Off

Instructor: _____ Date: _____

© 2015 Pearson Education, Inc.

Procedure 17-4:

Obtain Authorization from an Insurance Company for a Procedure

Objective: Obtain an authorization from an insurance carrier for a procedure correctly within the time limit set by the instructor.

Supplies: Patient insurance information (i.e., ID number, birthdate of the insured, name and telephone number for provider customer service at the insurance company); paper and pen; description of the procedure the doctor has prescribed, including Current Procedural Terminology (CPT) code; patient's diagnosis pertaining to the needed procedure; location where procedure is to be performed (e.g., office, outpatient surgery, inpatient hospitalization); date by which the procedure must be performed.

Affective Behaviors: Affective behaviors provide a professional approach to a skill that enhances the patient encounter. These behaviors may also display sensitivity to patients' rights, enhance communication, convey an understanding of laws and regulations, and/or provide an overall professional component to the medical assisting profession. Pay close attention to these skills, which appear in **bold, *italicized*** font.

Notes to the Student:

_____

_____

_____

_____

_____

_____

_____

Skills Assessment Requirements

Read and familiarize yourself with the procedure; complete the minimum practice requirements (MPRs). Document each MPR using proper charting technique. Complete each procedure within a reasonable amount of time, with a minimum of 85 percent accuracy.

© 2015 Pearson Education, Inc.

Name: _____

Date: _____

POINT VALUE ◆ = 3–6 points ★ = 7–9 points	PRACTICE TRIAL	GRADED TRIAL #1	GRADED TRIAL #2	NOTES:
1. ★ Write down the date and time of the call, the name of the insurance company, and the name of the insurance company representative on the phone.				
2. ◆ ***Warmly greet the insurance company representative and state your name and your office's/physician's name.***				
3. ◆ Give the insurance company representative the name of the patient, the name of the insured, and the insured's ID number.				
4. ◆ Let the representative know what procedure your doctor has prescribed for the patient and the date by which the procedure must be performed.				
5. ◆ Provide the representative with any other requested information (e.g., procedure code, diagnosis code, and place where the procedure is to be performed).				
6. ★ Write down the authorization number the representative provides.				

© 2015 Pearson Education, Inc.

7. ★	Ask the representative if any supporting documentation (e.g., chart notes, operative report, laboratory report, or pathology report) will be needed with the CMS-1500 billing form. If so, write down the required documentation. ***Thank the representative and end the call.***				
8. ★	Keep all preceding information in the patient's file for reference in case the claim is not paid by the insurance carrier.				

© 2015 Pearson Education, Inc.

Name: _____

Date: _____

Document: Enter the appropriate information in the chart below.

Grading

Points Earned	_____		
Points Possible	_____	60	60
Percent Grade (Points Earned/Points Possible)	_____		
PASS:	_____	❑ YES ❑ NO ❑ N/A	❑ YES ❑ NO ❑ N/A

Instructor Sign-Off

Instructor: _____ **Date:** _____

© 2015 Pearson Education, Inc.

Procedure 17-5:

Handle a Denied Insurance Claim

Objective: To handle a denied insurance claim in the time frame designated by the instructor.

Supplies: Patient insurance information (i.e., ID number, birthdate of the insured, name and provider customer service telephone number of insurance company); paper and pen; copy of the explanation of benefits (EOB) received; description of the procedure the doctor has performed, including CPT code; patient's diagnosis pertaining to the procedure performed; the location where the procedure was performed (e.g., office, outpatient surgery, inpatient hospitalization); date the procedure was performed; any documentation of the service having been preauthorized by the office.

Notes to the Student:

_____

_____

_____

_____

_____

_____

_____

Skills Assessment Requirements

Read and familiarize yourself with the procedure; complete the minimum practice requirements (MPRs). Document each MPR using proper charting technique. Complete each procedure within a reasonable amount of time, with a minimum of 85 percent accuracy.

© 2015 Pearson Education, Inc.

Name: _____

Date: _____

POINT VALUE ◆ = 3–6 points ★ = 7–9 points		PRACTICE TRIAL	GRADED TRIAL #1	GRADED TRIAL #2	NOTES:
1. ◆	Organize all materials.				
2. ◆	Call the insurance company's provider customer service phone number as listed on the patient's insurance identification card.				
3. ◆	Write down the date and time of the telephone call, the number called, and the name of the customer service representative on the phone.				
4. ◆	Self-identify to the customer service representative, and provide the patient's identification number and date of service.				
5. ◆	If the service was preauthorized, give that information to the customer service representative.				
6. ◆	Ask the customer service representative why the procedure was not paid as anticipated.				
7. ◆	If there was an error in processing the service for payment, ask the customer service representative if any other information is needed to process the claim correctly. Ask the customer service representative when the office can expect payment for the procedure.				
8. ◆	If the customer service representative says the claim was correctly processed, request the reason for the denial.				

© 2015 Pearson Education, Inc.

9. ◆	If the reason for the denial was lack of supporting documentation, ask the customer service representative if faxing the information is a solution. If the answer is yes, get the customer service representative's direct fax line and fax the needed documentation.				
10. ◆	If the reason for the denial requires an appeal be filed, ask the customer service representative to explain the insurance company's process for appeals.				
11. ◆	Write down any pertinent information, such as where to mail the appeal and what information the appeal should contain.				
12. ◆	Call the patient with the findings and get the patient involved as needed.				

© 2015 Pearson Education, Inc.

Name: _____

Date: _____

Document: Enter the appropriate information in the chart below.

Grading

Points Earned	_____		
Points Possible	_____	72	72
Percent Grade (Points Earned/Points Possible)	_____		
PASS:	_____	❏ YES ❏ NO ❏ N/A	❏ YES ❏ NO ❏ N/A

Instructor Sign-Off

Instructor: _____ **Date:** _____

© 2015 Pearson Education, Inc.

Procedure 17-6:

Abstract Data to Complete a Paper CMS-1500 Claim Form

Objective: Abstract data from the medical record to complete a CMS-1500 Claim Form.

Supplies: Klaus Davies patient registration form, insurance ID card, encounter form, Capital City Medical fee schedule, instructions on completing the CMS-1500 Claim Form, blank CMS-1500 form, black ink pen, calculator.

Notes to the Student:

_____

_____

_____

_____

_____

_____

Skills Assessment Requirements

Read and familiarize yourself with the procedure; complete the minimum practice requirements (MPRs). Document each MPR using proper charting technique. Complete each procedure within a reasonable amount of time, with a minimum of 85 percent accuracy.

© 2015 Pearson Education, Inc.

Name: _____

Date: _____

POINT VALUE ◆ = 3–6 points ★ = 7–9 points	PRACTICE TRIAL	GRADED TRIAL #1	GRADED TRIAL #2	NOTES:
1. ◆ Enter the insurance company name and mailing address in the Carrier Area.				
2. ◆ Check the correct box in Item 1.				
3. ◆ Enter the insured's ID number in Item 1a.				
4. ◆ Enter the patient's name in Item 2, if different from the insured.				
5. ◆ Complete Item 3, using MMDDCCYY date format.				
6. ◆ Complete Item 4.				
7. ◆ Leave Item 5 blank because it is the same as Item 7.				
8. ◆ Complete Item 6.				
9. ◆ Complete Item 7. Note there are three lines of information to complete.				
10. ◆ Leave Item 8 blank.				
11. ◆ Leave Item 9a to 9d blank because there is no secondary insurance.				
12. ◆ Complete Item 10a, 10b, and 10c.				
13. ◆ Leave Item 10d blank.				
14. ◆ Enter the group number in Item 11.				
15. ◆ Complete Item 11a, using MMDDCCYY date format.				
16. ◆ Leave Item 11b blank.				
17. ◆ Enter the insurance plan name in Item 11c.				
18. ◆ Mark NO in Item 11d.				
19. ◆ Enter "SOF" in Item 12.				
20. ◆ Enter "SOF" in Item 13.				

© 2015 Pearson Education, Inc.

21. ◆	Leave Item 14 to Item 19 blank.				
22. ◆	Mark NO in Item 20.				
23. ★	Enter the first diagnosis code in Item 21, line A.				
24. ★	Enter the second diagnosis code in Item 21, line B.				
25. ◆	Leave Item 22 to Item 23 blank.				
26. ◆	In Item 24A, line 1, enter the date of service in both the FROM and TO fields.				
27. ◆	Enter the code number for place of service in Item 24B.				
28. ◆	Leave Item 24C blank.				
29. ★	Enter the first CPT code in Item 24D.				
30. ★	In Item 24E, enter "A B" to designate that both diagnoses 1 and 2 relate to this service.				
31. ★	Look on the encounter form to find the description for CPT code 99231. Then look on the fee schedule to find the fee for this service and enter it in Item 24F.				
32. ◆	Enter 1 for units in Item 24G.				
33. ◆	Leave blank Item 24H and Item 24I.				
34. ◆	Enter the physician's NPI number on the unshaded portion of 24J. You will find the number on the encounter form.				
35. ◆	Repeat these steps for lines 2 through 6. In Item 24E be certain you designate the correct diagnosis reference for each service, as some lines will be only "A" or only "B."				

© 2015 Pearson Education, Inc.

36. ◆	When all services are completed, enter the EIN in Item 25 and mark X in the appropriate box. You will find this information on the patient registration form.				
37. ◆	Enter the patient's account number in Item 26. You will find this on the patient registration form.				
38. ◆	Mark YES in Item 27.				
39. ◆	Add up the total charges in column 24F. Write the total in Item 28.				
40. ◆	Leave Item 29 and Item 30 blank.				
41. ◆	Enter the physician's signature, credentials, and the date in Item 31. Be certain to stay within the lines of the box.				
42. ◆	In Item 33, enter the clinic's phone number in the top right corner.				
43. ◆	Enter the clinic's name and address in Item 33.				
44. ◆	Enter the clinic's NPI number in Item 33a.				
45. ◆	Leave Item 33b blank.				
46. ◆	Proofread your work. Check all spelling and numbers against your source documents.				
47. ◆	Check your claim against the sample CMS-1500 form in Figure 17-20 of the student text.				

© 2015 Pearson Education, Inc.

Name: _____

Date: _____

Document: Enter the appropriate information in the chart below.

Grading

Points Earned	_____		
Points Possible	_____	297	297
Percent Grade (Points Earned/Points Possible)	_____		
PASS:	_____	❏ YES ❏ NO ❏ N/A	❏ YES ❏ NO ❏ N/A

Instructor Sign-Off

Instructor: _____ **Date:** _____

Name: _____

Date: _____

Procedure 17-7:

Complete a Computerized Insurance Claim Form

Objective: Complete a computerized insurance claim form correctly within the time limit set by the instructor.

Supplies: Computer with medical billing software, patient medical chart, fee slip for patient's visit.

Notes to the Student:

_____

_____

_____

_____

_____

_____

Skills Assessment Requirements

Read and familiarize yourself with the procedure; complete the minimum practice requirements (MPRs). Document each MPR using proper charting technique. Complete each procedure within a reasonable amount of time, with a minimum of 85 percent accuracy.

© 2015 Pearson Education, Inc.

Name: _____

Date: _____

POINT VALUE ◆ = 3–6 points ★ = 7–9 points		PRACTICE TRIAL	GRADED TRIAL #1	GRADED TRIAL #2	NOTES:
1. ◆	Choose the patient's account ledger in the computer billing software.				
2. ★	Verify that the fee slip is for the patient with the account opened on the computer.				
3. ◆	Enter the charges and coding as appropriate.				
4. ◆	Complete the patient insurance information field.				
5. ◆	Enter the patient's information, including address, telephone number, and birthdate.				
6. ◆	Enter the insured's information, including address, telephone number, and birthdate.				
7. ◆	Enter the patient's relationship to the insured.				
8. ◆	Enter the insured's identification and group number.				
9. ◆	Check the appropriate box to indicate the patient has authorized the release of information to the insurance company.				
10. ◆	Check the appropriate box to indicate the patient has assigned the benefits (payment) to the provider.				
11. ◆	Check the appropriate boxes to indicate if the visit was related to an accident.				
12. ◆	If the visit was due to an accident, enter the accident's date.				

© 2015 Pearson Education, Inc.

13. ◆	Enter any information regarding a referring physician, if applicable.				
14. ◆	Enter any information regarding the patient's need for hospitalization for these charges, if applicable.				
15. ◆	Enter the treating provider's name, address, telephone number, national provider identification (NPI) number, and Internal Revenue Service (IRS) tax identification number.				
16. ◆	Enter information regarding the facility where the services were performed if not performed in the provider's office.				
17. ★	Check the appropriate box to indicate the provider accepts assignment.				
18. ◆	Print the patient's insurance claim form.				
19. ◆	Review the form for accuracy and completeness.				
20. ◆	Send the claim to the insurance company.				

© 2015 Pearson Education, Inc.

Name: _____

Date: _____

Document: Enter the appropriate information in the chart below.

Grading

Points Earned	_____		
Points Possible	_____	114	114
Percent Grade (Points Earned/Points Possible)	_____		
PASS:	_____	❑ YES ❑ NO ❑ N/A	❑ YES ❑ NO ❑ N/A

Instructor Sign-Off

Instructor: _____ **Date:** _____

© 2015 Pearson Education, Inc.

Procedure 18-1:

Perform Diagnostic Coding Using ICD-10-CM

Objective: Perform diagnostic coding correctly within the time limit set by the instructor.

Supplies: Patient's medical chart, current ICD-10-CM coding manual, superbill with doctor's written diagnosis.

Notes to the Student:

_____

_____

_____

_____

_____

_____

_____

Skills Assessment Requirements

Read and familiarize yourself with the procedure; complete the minimum practice requirements (MPRs). Document each MPR using proper charting technique. Complete each procedure within a reasonable amount of time, with a minimum of 85 percent accuracy.

Name: _____

Date: _____

POINT VALUE ◆ = 3–6 points ★ = 7–9 points		PRACTICE TRIAL	GRADED TRIAL #1	GRADED TRIAL #2	NOTES:
1. ◆	Locate the patient's diagnostic code(s) on the superbill or in the chart notes.				
2. ★	Verify that the diagnostic code(s) or description on the superbill is documented in the patient's chart.				
3. ◆	Look in the Index of the ICD-10-CM coding manual to find the Main Term, subterm, and preliminary diagnosis code.				
4. ◆	Look up the preliminary code(s) in the Tabular List. Confirm that the written description matches the chart notes. If in doubt, check with the physician.				
5. ◆	Read and apply the conventions in the Tabular List.				
6. ◆	Assign the code for each diagnosis, beginning with the appropriate first-listed diagnosis.				

© 2015 Pearson Education, Inc.

Name: _____

Date: _____

Document: Enter the appropriate information in the chart below.

Grading

Points Earned	_____		
Points Possible	_____	36	36
Percent Grade (Points Earned/Points Possible)	_____		
PASS:	_____	❏ YES ❏ NO ❏ N/A	❏ YES ❏ NO ❏ N/A

Instructor Sign-Off

Instructor: _____   **Date:** _____

© 2015 Pearson Education, Inc.

Procedure 19-1:

Code for a Procedure

Objective: Assign a procedure code correctly within the time limit set by the instructor.

Supplies: CPT coding manual, superbill/encounter form, patient's chart.

Affective Behaviors: Affective behaviors provide a professional approach to a skill that enhances the patient encounter. These behaviors may also display sensitivity to patients' rights, enhance communication, convey an understanding of laws and regulations, and/or provide an overall professional component to the medical assisting profession. Pay close attention to these skills, which appear in **_bold, italicized_** font.

Notes to the Student:

_____

_____

_____

_____

_____

_____

_____

Skills Assessment Requirements

Read and familiarize yourself with the procedure; complete the minimum practice requirements (MPRs). Document each MPR using proper charting technique. Complete each procedure within a reasonable amount of time, with a minimum of 85 percent accuracy.

© 2015 Pearson Education, Inc.

POINT VALUE ◆ = 3–6 points ★ = 7–9 points		PRACTICE TRIAL	GRADED TRIAL #1	GRADED TRIAL #2	NOTES:
1. ◆	On the superbill, locate the procedure code the physician has circled.				
2. ◆	Identify the primary and secondary services or procedures performed, as stated in the medical record.				
3. ◆	Locate the Main Term in the Index.				
4. ★	Review any modifying terms or instructional notes associated with the Main Term.				
5. ◆	Identify the preliminary code(s) associated with the most appropriate modifying term(s).				
6. ◆	Locate the preliminary code(s) in the Tabular List.				
7. ★	Interpret the conventions used in the Tabular List.				
8. ★	**Select the code with the highest level of specificity.**				
9. ◆	Review the code for appropriate bundling, add-on codes, and quantity.				
10. ★	Determine if modifiers are required.				
11. ★	Verify the final code against documentation.				
12. ◆	Assign the code.				

© 2015 Pearson Education, Inc.

Name: _____

Date: _____

Document: Enter the appropriate information in the chart below.

Grading

Points Earned	_____		
Points Possible	_____	87	87
Percent Grade (Points Earned/Points Possible)	_____		
PASS:	_____	❏ YES ❏ NO ❏ N/A	❏ YES ❏ NO ❏ N/A

Instructor Sign-Off

Instructor: _____ **Date:** _____

© 2015 Pearson Education, Inc.

Name: _____

Date: _____

Procedure 20-1:

Prepare an Accounts Receivable Trial Balance

Objective: Correctly prepare an accounts receivable trial balance.

Supplies: Patient accounts in computerized format, computer, fee slips for services rendered to the patients for the day, calculator, pen.

Notes to the Student:

_____

_____

_____

_____

_____

_____

_____

Skills Assessment Requirements

Read and familiarize yourself with the procedure; complete the minimum practice requirements (MPRs). Document each MPR using proper charting technique. Complete each procedure within a reasonable amount of time, with a minimum of 85 percent accuracy.

Name: _____

Date: _____

POINT VALUE ◆ = 3–6 points ★ = 7–9 points		PRACTICE TRIAL	GRADED TRIAL #1	GRADED TRIAL #2	NOTES:
1. ★	Calculate the total of the charges on the fee slips for the day.				
2. ★	Using the computer, calculate the total of the charges posted to patient accounts for the day.				
3. ◆	Compare the total of the charges from the fee slips to the total of the charges in the computer.				
4. ◆	If the balances do not match, calculate the totals a second time to verify you added them correctly.				
5. ◆	If the balances continue to differ, go through the fee slips to see where the error in entry has occurred.				
6. ◆	Correct the entry error and calculate the totals again.				
7. ◆	If the balances continue to differ, go through the above steps until they match.				

© 2015 Pearson Education, Inc.

Name: _____

Date: _____

Document: Enter the appropriate information in the chart below.

Grading

Points Earned	_____		
Points Possible	_____	48	48
Percent Grade (Points Earned/Points Possible)	_____		
PASS:	_____	❏ YES ❏ NO ❏ N/A	❏ YES ❏ NO ❏ N/A

Instructor Sign-Off

Instructor: _____ **Date:** _____

© 2015 Pearson Education, Inc.

Procedure 20-2:

Explain Professional Fees to a Patient

Objective: Explain the physician's professional fees to a patient correctly within the time limit set by the instructor.

Supplies: Patient medical record, copy of office fee schedule, blue or black pen, payment contract.

Affective Behaviors: Affective behaviors provide a professional approach to a skill that enhances the patient encounter. These behaviors may also display sensitivity to patients' rights, enhance communication, convey an understanding of laws and regulations, and/or provide an overall professional component to the medical assisting profession. Pay close attention to these skills, which appear in **bold, italicized** font.

Notes to the Student:

_____

_____

_____

_____

_____

_____

_____

Skills Assessment Requirements

Read and familiarize yourself with the procedure; complete the minimum practice requirements (MPRs). Document each MPR using proper charting technique. Complete each procedure within a reasonable amount of time, with a minimum of 85 percent accuracy.

© 2015 Pearson Education, Inc.

Name: _____

Date: _____

POINT VALUE ◆ = 3–6 points ★ = 7–9 points		PRACTICE TRIAL	GRADED TRIAL #1	GRADED TRIAL #2	NOTES:
1. ◆	**Find a private location to** sit with the patient.				
2. ◆	Explain to the patient the procedure the physician has prescribed.				
3. ◆	Explain to the patient the fee for the procedure.				
4. ◆	Explain to the patient any insurance coverage for the fee.				
5. ◆	**With a professional tone, explain to the patient the payment amount and deadline. Try to remain sensitive to the patient's financial situation.**				
6. ◆	Secure an agreement from the patient about the payment date.				
7. ◆	Enter the payment agreement and arrangements on the payment contract. **Ask the patient if he or she has any questions prior to signing the contract.**				
8. ★	On the payment contract, obtain the patient's signature and sign as the witness.				
9. ◆	Answer any questions the patient may have about the fee or the procedure.				
10. ★	Place the payment agreement in the patient's financial record.				

© 2015 Pearson Education, Inc.

Name: _____

Date: _____

Document: Enter the appropriate information in the chart below.

Grading

Points Earned	_____		
Points Possible	_____	66	66
Percent Grade (Points Earned/Points Possible)	_____		
PASS:	_____	❏ YES ❏ NO ❏ N/A	❏ YES ❏ NO ❏ N/A

Instructor Sign-Off

Instructor: _____   **Date:** _____

© 2015 Pearson Education, Inc.

Procedure 20-3:

Call a Patient Regarding an Overdue Account

Objective: Call a patient regarding an overdue account correctly within the time limit set by the instructor.

Supplies: Telephone, electronic patient ledger, blue or black ink pen.

Affective Behaviors: Affective behaviors provide a professional approach to a skill that enhances the patient encounter. These behaviors may also display sensitivity to patients' rights, enhance communication, convey an understanding of laws and regulations, and/or provide an overall professional component to the medical assisting profession. Pay close attention to these skills, which appear in **_bold, italicized_** font.

Notes to the Student:

_____

_____

_____

_____

_____

_____

Skills Assessment Requirements

Read and familiarize yourself with the procedure; complete the minimum practice requirements (MPRs). Document each MPR using proper charting technique. Complete each procedure within a reasonable amount of time, with a minimum of 85 percent accuracy.

© 2015 Pearson Education, Inc.

POINT VALUE ◆ = 3–6 points ★ = 7–9 points		PRACTICE TRIAL	GRADED TRIAL #1	GRADED TRIAL #2	NOTES:
1. ◆	Dial the patient's home telephone number.				
2. ★	If you reach the patient, **using a professional and nonconfrontational voice:** **a.** Identify yourself and the name of your clinic and state the reason for the call. **b.** Ask the patient when payment on the outstanding bill will be made. **c.** If the patient agrees to pay via credit card, take the credit card information over the telephone, verify the amount to be charged, and mail the patient a receipt. **d.** If the patient agrees to mail payment to the office, secure a date by which the payment is to be received and note the date in the patient's electronic billing ledger. **e.** If the patient expresses an inability to make a payment at this time, secure a date by which the patient expects to be able to make a payment and note the date in the patient's electronic billing ledger. **Express thanks to the patient for assisting in resolving the matter.**				

© 2015 Pearson Education, Inc.

3. ◆	If unable to reach the patient, leave a message that discloses no personal information about the patient's care in the office.				
4. ★	Note the message in the patient's electronic billing ledger.				

Document: Enter the appropriate information in the chart below.

Grading

Points Earned	_____		
Points Possible	_____	30	30
Percent Grade (Points Earned/Points Possible)	_____		
PASS:	_____	❏ YES ❏ NO ❏ N/A	❏ YES ❏ NO ❏ N/A

Instructor Sign-Off

Instructor: _____   Date: _____

© 2015 Pearson Education, Inc.

Procedure 20-4:

Send a Patient Billing Statement

Objective: Send a patient billing statement correctly within the time limit set by the instructor.

Supplies: Computer with medical billing software, printer.

Notes to the Student:

_____

_____

_____

_____

_____

_____

_____

Skills Assessment Requirements

Read and familiarize yourself with the procedure; complete the minimum practice requirements (MPRs). Document each MPR using proper charting technique. Complete each procedure within a reasonable amount of time, with a minimum of 85 percent accuracy.

© 2015 Pearson Education, Inc.

Name: _____

Date: _____

POINT VALUE ◆ = 3–6 points ★ = 7–9 points	PRACTICE TRIAL	GRADED TRIAL #1	GRADED TRIAL #2	NOTES:
1. ◆ Once printed, verify the information on the bill is correct.				
2. ◆ Place a copy of the bill into an envelope.				
3. ◆ Stamp the envelope and place it in the mail.				

© 2015 Pearson Education, Inc.

Name: _____

Date: _____

Document: Enter the appropriate information in the chart below.

Grading

Points Earned	_____		
Points Possible	_____	18	18
Percent Grade (Points Earned/Points Possible)	_____		
PASS:	_____	❏ YES ❏ NO ❏ N/A	❏ YES ❏ NO ❏ N/A

Instructor Sign-Off

Instructor: _____   **Date:** _____

© 2015 Pearson Education, Inc.

Procedure 20-5:

Post a Nonsufficient Funds Check

Objective: Post an NSF check correctly within the time limit set by the instructor.

Supplies: Check returned due to NSF, computer with medical billing software.

Notes to the Student:

_____

_____

_____

_____

_____

_____

_____

Skills Assessment Requirements

Read and familiarize yourself with the procedure; complete the minimum practice requirements (MPRs). Document each MPR using proper charting technique. Complete each procedure within a reasonable amount of time, with a minimum of 85 percent accuracy.

© 2015 Pearson Education, Inc.

Name: _____

Date: _____

POINT VALUE ◆ = 3–6 points ★ = 7–9 points		PRACTICE TRIAL	GRADED TRIAL #1	GRADED TRIAL #2	NOTES:
1. ◆	Verify that you have located the correct patient in the medical billing system.				
2. ◆	Enter the NSF check and any fees into the patient's account.				
3. ★	*Notify the patient via phone that the check was returned. Indicate any corresponding fees.*				
4. ◆	Secure a date by which a replacement payment will be received.				
5. ◆	In the patient's ledger, note the outcome of the conversation.				

© 2015 Pearson Education, Inc.

Name: _____

Date: _____

Document: Enter the appropriate information in the chart below.

Grading

Points Earned	_____		
Points Possible	_____	33	33
Percent Grade (Points Earned/Points Possible)	_____		
PASS:	_____	❏ YES ❏ NO ❏ N/A	❏ YES ❏ NO ❏ N/A

Instructor Sign-Off

Instructor: _____ **Date:** _____

© 2015 Pearson Education, Inc.

Name: _____

Date: _____

Procedure 20-6:

Post an Adjustment to a Patient Account

Objective: Post an adjustment to a patient account correctly within the time limit set by the instructor.

Supplies: Medical billing software.

Notes to the Student:

_____

_____

_____

_____

_____

_____

_____

Skills Assessment Requirements

Read and familiarize yourself with the procedure; complete the minimum practice requirements (MPRs). Document each MPR using proper charting technique. Complete each procedure within a reasonable amount of time, with a minimum of 85 percent accuracy.

© 2015 Pearson Education, Inc.

Name: _____

Date: _____

POINT VALUE ◆ = 3–6 points ★ = 7–9 points		PRACTICE TRIAL	GRADED TRIAL #1	GRADED TRIAL #2	NOTES:
1. ★	Locate the correct patient ledger in the computer.				
2. ★	Enter the adjustment as a debit or a credit.				
3. ★	In the patient's financial record, note the reason for the adjustment.				

© 2015 Pearson Education, Inc.

Name: _____

Date: _____

Document: Enter the appropriate information in the chart below.

Grading

Points Earned	_____		
Points Possible	_____	27	27
Percent Grade (Points Earned/Points Possible)	_____		
PASS:	_____	❏ YES ❏ NO ❏ N/A	❏ YES ❏ NO ❏ N/A

Instructor Sign-Off

Instructor: _____ **Date:** _____

© 2015 Pearson Education, Inc.

Procedure 20-7:

Post a Collection Agency Payment

Objective: Post a collection agency payment correctly within the time limit set by the instructor.

Supplies: Calculator, computer, collection agency payment.

Notes to the Student:

_____

_____

_____

_____

_____

_____

_____

Skills Assessment Requirements

Read and familiarize yourself with the procedure; complete the minimum practice requirements (MPRs). Document each MPR using proper charting technique. Complete each procedure within a reasonable amount of time, with a minimum of 85 percent accuracy.

© 2015 Pearson Education, Inc.

Name: _____

Date: _____

POINT VALUE ◆ = 3–6 points ★ = 7–9 points	PRACTICE TRIAL	GRADED TRIAL #1	GRADED TRIAL #2	NOTES:
1. ◆ Find the patient's account in the computer.				
2. ◆ Verify that the patient account is correct.				
3. ★ Post the payment, choosing "collection payment" as the payment source.				
4. ◆ If applicable, enter any adjustment due to collection agency fee.				
5. ◆ Verify the payment amount and adjustment.				
6. ★ Save all changes.				

© 2015 Pearson Education, Inc.

Name: _____

Date: _____

Document: Enter the appropriate information in the chart below.

Grading

Points Earned	_____		
Points Possible	_____	42	42
Percent Grade (Points Earned/Points Possible)	_____		
PASS:	_____	❏ YES ❏ NO ❏ N/A	❏ YES ❏ NO ❏ N/A

Instructor Sign-Off

Instructor: _____   **Date:** _____

© 2015 Pearson Education, Inc.

Procedure 20-8:

Process a Patient Refund

Objective: Process a refund to a patient correctly within the time limit set by the instructor.

Supplies: Computer with medical billing software.

Notes to the Student:

_____

_____

_____

_____

_____

_____

_____

Skills Assessment Requirements

Read and familiarize yourself with the procedure; complete the minimum practice requirements (MPRs). Document each MPR using proper charting technique. Complete each procedure within a reasonable amount of time, with a minimum of 85 percent accuracy.

© 2015 Pearson Education, Inc.

Name: _____

Date: _____

POINT VALUE ◆ = 3–6 points ★ = 7–9 points		PRACTICE TRIAL	GRADED TRIAL #1	GRADED TRIAL #2	NOTES:
1. ◆	Locate the proper patient ledger in the billing software.				
2. ◆	Enter the refund amount.				
3. ◆	Choose the adjustment code for "Refund to Patient."				
4. ★	Obtain a refund check from the physician or office manager.				
5. ◆	Send the refund check to the patient.				
6. ★	In the patient ledger, note the party receiving the refund and the number of the refund check.				

© 2015 Pearson Education, Inc.

Name: _____

Date: _____

Document: Enter the appropriate information in the chart below.

Grading

Points Earned	_____		
Points Possible	_____	42	42
Percent Grade (Points Earned/Points Possible)	_____		
PASS:	_____	❏ YES ❏ NO ❏ N/A	❏ YES ❏ NO ❏ N/A

Instructor Sign-Off

Instructor: _____ **Date:** _____

Name: _____

Date: _____

Procedure 20-9:

Process an Insurance Company Overpayment

Objective: Process a refund to an insurance company correctly within the time limit set by the instructor.

Supplies: Computer with medical billing software, copies of insurance companies' explanation of benefits.

Notes to the Student:

_____

_____

_____

_____

_____

_____

_____

Skills Assessment Requirements

Read and familiarize yourself with the procedure; complete the minimum practice requirements (MPRs). Document each MPR using proper charting technique. Complete each procedure within a reasonable amount of time, with a minimum of 85 percent accuracy.

© 2015 Pearson Education, Inc.

POINT VALUE ◆ = 3–6 points ★ = 7–9 points		PRACTICE TRIAL	GRADED TRIAL #1	GRADED TRIAL #2	NOTES:
1. ◆	Using the insurance companies' explanations of benefits, determine which company is the patient's primary insurance carrier and which is secondary.				
2. ◆	Find the appropriate patient ledger in the computer.				
3. ◆	Using the appropriate code, enter the refund to the insurance company.				
4. ★	Obtain a refund check from the physician or office manager.				
5. ★	Send a note to the insurance company explaining the reason for the refund, as well as copies of the primary and secondary insurance companies' explanations of benefits.				

© 2015 Pearson Education, Inc.

Name: _____

Date: _____

Document: Enter the appropriate information in the chart below.

Grading

Points Earned	_____		
Points Possible	_____	36	36
Percent Grade (Points Earned/Points Possible)	_____		
PASS:	_____	❑ YES ❑ NO ❑ N/A	❑ YES ❑ NO ❑ N/A

Instructor Sign-Off

Instructor: _____   **Date:** _____

© 2015 Pearson Education, Inc.

Procedure 21-1:

Create a New Employee Record

Objective: Create a new employee record correctly within the time limit set by the instructor.

Supplies: Pen, paper, employee file, copy machine.

Notes to the Student:

_____

_____

_____

_____

_____

_____

_____

Skills Assessment Requirements

Read and familiarize yourself with the procedure; complete the minimum practice requirements (MPRs). Document each MPR using proper charting technique. Complete each procedure within a reasonable amount of time, with a minimum of 85 percent accuracy.

© 2015 Pearson Education, Inc.

POINT VALUE ◆ = 3–6 points ★ = 7–9 points		PRACTICE TRIAL	GRADED TRIAL #1	GRADED TRIAL #2	NOTES:
1. ◆	Ask the new employee to bring the following items with him on his first day of employment: • Picture identification or other proof of ability to work in the United States • Social Security card • Copies of any certifications or professional licenses				
2. ★	Photocopy any documents the employee has brought for the employee record.				
3. ◆	Give the employee a W-4 IRS form to complete to indicate the number of exemptions to be claimed.				
4. ◆	Place the employee's résumé and application into the employee record.				
5. ◆	Give the employee an I-9 form to complete to verify citizenship.				

© 2015 Pearson Education, Inc.

Document: Enter the appropriate information in the chart below.

Grading

Points Earned	_____		
Points Possible	_____	33	33
Percent Grade (Points Earned/Points Possible)	_____		
PASS:	_____	❏ YES ❏ NO ❏ N/A	❏ YES ❏ NO ❏ N/A

Instructor Sign-Off

Instructor: _____ **Date:** _____

© 2015 Pearson Education, Inc.

Name: _____

Date: _____

Procedure 21-2:

Calculate an Employee's Payroll

Objective: Calculate the amount of an employee's payroll correctly within the time limit set by the instructor.

Supplies: Calculator, employee's W-4 form, IRS Circular E list of federal tax deduction amounts, record of number of hours the employee worked, employee's payroll record.

Affective Behaviors: Affective behaviors provide a professional approach to a skill that enhances the patient encounter. These behaviors may also display sensitivity to patients' rights, enhance communication, convey an understanding of laws and regulations, and/or provide an overall professional component to the medical assisting profession. Pay close attention to these skills, which appear in **bold, *italicized*** font.

Notes to the Student:

_____

_____

_____

_____

_____

_____

_____

Skills Assessment Requirements

Read and familiarize yourself with the procedure; complete the minimum practice requirements (MPRs). Document each MPR using proper charting technique. Complete each procedure within a reasonable amount of time, with a minimum of 85 percent accuracy.

© 2015 Pearson Education, Inc.

Name: _____

Date: _____

POINT VALUE ◆ = 3–6 points ★ = 7–9 points		PRACTICE TRIAL	GRADED TRIAL #1	GRADED TRIAL #2	NOTES:
1. ★	Calculate the number of hours the employee worked during the payroll period.				
2. ◆	For an hourly employee, calculate the employee's gross wage by multiplying the number of hours worked in the payroll period by the employee's hourly wage. ***Keep in mind that the employee's wage is confidential and should never be discussed with anyone other than the employee.***				
3. ◆	If the employee worked any overtime hours, first multiply the employee's hourly wage by 1.5 and then multiply that amount by the employee's overtime hours.				
4. ◆	Consult the employee's W-4 form to determine filing status (i.e., married or single) and the number of deductions.				
5. ◆	Consult the IRS Circular E form to determine the amount to be withheld from the employee's gross wages.				
6. ★	Deduct the federal withholding tax found on the Circular E form from the employee's gross payroll.				
7. ◆	Multiply the employee's gross payroll amount by 6.2 percent to determine the FICA (Social Security) to withhold from the employee's payroll.				

© 2015 Pearson Education, Inc.

8. ◆	Multiply the employee's gross payroll amount by 1.45 percent to determine the Medicare tax to withhold from the employee's payroll.				
9. ★	Consult the employee's file to determine any other deductions (e.g., health insurance or retirement contributions) to withhold from the employee's payroll.				
10. ◆	Determine the net payroll by subtracting all deductions from the gross payroll.				

© 2015 Pearson Education, Inc.

Name: _____

Date: _____

Document: Enter the appropriate information in the chart below.

Grading

Points Earned	_____		
Points Possible	_____	69	69
Percent Grade (Points Earned/Points Possible)	_____		
PASS:	_____	❏ YES ❏ NO ❏ N/A	❏ YES ❏ NO ❏ N/A

Instructor Sign-Off

Instructor: _____ Date: _____

© 2015 Pearson Education, Inc.

Procedure 21-3:

Write Checks to Pay Bills

Objective: Write checks in payment of office bills correctly within the time limit set by the instructor.

Supplies: Office checkbook register, bills to be paid, blue or black pen, calculator.

Notes to the Student:

_____

_____

_____

_____

_____

_____

_____

Skills Assessment Requirements

Read and familiarize yourself with the procedure; complete the minimum practice requirements (MPRs). Document each MPR using proper charting technique. Complete each procedure within a reasonable amount of time, with a minimum of 85 percent accuracy.

© 2015 Pearson Education, Inc.

POINT VALUE ◆ = 3–6 points ★ = 7–9 points		PRACTICE TRIAL	GRADED TRIAL #1	GRADED TRIAL #2	NOTES:
1. ◆	Verify the bill is accurate and that the supplies or services were received.				
2. ◆	Determine if the company offers a discount if the bill is paid by a certain date. If so, pay the bill by the discount due date to obtain the discount.				
3. ★	Complete the check, providing the date, name of the vendor or supplier, and check amount.				
4. ◆	On the invoice, write the date, check number, and payment amount.				
5. ◆	File the invoice.				
6. ★	Give the check to the physician or office manager for signature.				
7. ◆	In the checkbook register, note the payment category, date, and amount of the check.				

© 2015 Pearson Education, Inc.

Name: _____

Date: _____

Document: Enter the appropriate information in the chart below.

Grading

Points Earned	_____		
Points Possible	_____	48	48
Percent Grade (Points Earned/Points Possible)	_____		
PASS:	_____	❏ YES ❏ NO ❏ N/A	❏ YES ❏ NO ❏ N/A

Instructor Sign-Off

Instructor: _____   **Date:** _____

© 2015 Pearson Education, Inc.

Name: _____

Date: _____

Procedure 21-4:

Pay an Office Supply Invoice

Objective: Pay an office supply invoice correctly within the time limit set by the instructor.

Supplies: Office supply invoice, office checkbook and checkbook register, blue or black pen, calculator.

Notes to the Student:

_____

_____

_____

_____

_____

_____

_____

Skills Assessment Requirements

Read and familiarize yourself with the procedure; complete the minimum practice requirements (MPRs). Document each MPR using proper charting technique. Complete each procedure within a reasonable amount of time, with a minimum of 85 percent accuracy.

© 2015 Pearson Education, Inc.

Name: _____

Date: _____

POINT VALUE ◆ = 3–6 points ★ = 7–9 points		PRACTICE TRIAL	GRADED TRIAL #1	GRADED TRIAL #2	NOTES:
1. ◆	Verify that the supplies on the invoice were received, that inventory was taken of the supplies, and that the supplies were distributed in the office appropriately.				
2. ◆	Determine whether the supplier offers a discount if the bill is paid by a certain date. If so, pay the bill by the discount due date to obtain the discount.				
3. ★	Write a check for the supplies, providing the date, supplier name, and check amount.				
4. ★	Give the check to the physician or office manager for signature.				
5. ◆	In the office checkbook register, note the payment, including the supply category, the date, and the amount of the check.				
6. ◆	Mail the payment to the supplier.				

© 2015 Pearson Education, Inc.

Name: _____

Date: _____

Document: Enter the appropriate information in the chart below.

Grading

Points Earned	_____		
Points Possible	_____	42	42
Percent Grade (Points Earned/Points Possible)	_____		
PASS:	_____	❑ YES ❑ NO ❑ N/A	❑ YES ❑ NO ❑ N/A

Instructor Sign-Off

Instructor: _____   **Date:** _____

© 2015 Pearson Education, Inc.

Procedure 21-5:

Complete a Deposit Slip

Objective: Fill out a deposit slip correctly within the time limit set by the instructor.

Supplies: Calculator, deposit slip, printout from the electronic or manual billing system showing amount received for the day, pen, endorsement stamp.

Affective Behaviors: Affective behaviors provide a professional approach to a skill that enhances the patient encounter. These behaviors may also display sensitivity to patients' rights, enhance communication, convey an understanding of laws and regulations, and/or provide an overall professional component to the medical assisting profession. Pay close attention to these skills, which appear in **_bold, italicized_** font.

Notes to the Student:

_____

_____

_____

_____

_____

_____

Skills Assessment Requirements

Read and familiarize yourself with the procedure; complete the minimum practice requirements (MPRs). Document each MPR using proper charting technique. Complete each procedure within a reasonable amount of time, with a minimum of 85 percent accuracy.

© 2015 Pearson Education, Inc.

POINT VALUE ◆ = 3–6 points ★ = 7–9 points		PRACTICE TRIAL	GRADED TRIAL #1	GRADED TRIAL #2	NOTES:
1. ◆	**Perform this task out of view of patients, such as in a back office.** Check to see that all checks have been properly endorsed.				
2. ◆	Total all cash receipts.				
3. ◆	On the line marked "cash" on the deposit slip, list the cash receipt total.				
4. ◆	On the deposit slip, list each check individually by bank routing number or name of the patient or insurance company.				
5. ◆	Total the checks.				
6. ◆	On the appropriate line of the deposit slip, list the check total.				
7. ★	Total the checks and cash.				
8. ◆	On the appropriate line of the deposit slip, list the checks and cash total. **Double-check calculations for errors.**				
9. ◆	Attach the deposit slip, cash, and checks with a paper clip.				
10. ◆	Place the paper clipped deposit in an envelope.				
11. ◆	Take the deposit to the bank.				
12. ◆	Obtain a receipt.				
13. ◆	Return to the office.				
14. ★	Using the receipt, record the deposit amount in the clinic checkbook register.				

© 2015 Pearson Education, Inc.

Name: _____

Date: _____

Document: Enter the appropriate information in the chart below.

Grading

Points Earned	_____		
Points Possible	_____	90	90
Percent Grade (Points Earned/Points Possible)	_____		
PASS:	_____	❏ YES ❏ NO ❏ N/A	❏ YES ❏ NO ❏ N/A

Instructor Sign-Off

Instructor: _____ **Date:** _____

© 2015 Pearson Education, Inc.

Procedure 21-6:

Account for Petty Cash

Objective: Balance the petty cash fund correctly within the time limit set by the instructor.

Supplies: Petty cash record, receipts for petty cash purchases, blue or black ink pen, calculator.

Affective Behaviors: Affective behaviors provide a professional approach to a skill that enhances the patient encounter. These behaviors may also display sensitivity to patients' rights, enhance communication, convey an understanding of laws and regulations, and/or provide an overall professional component to the medical assisting profession. Pay close attention to these skills, which appear in **_bold, italicized_** font.

Notes to the Student: _____

_____
_____
_____
_____
_____
_____
_____

Skills Assessment Requirements

Read and familiarize yourself with the procedure; complete the minimum practice requirements (MPRs). Document each MPR using proper charting technique. Complete each procedure within a reasonable amount of time, with a minimum of 85 percent accuracy.

© 2015 Pearson Education, Inc.

Name: _____

Date: _____

POINT VALUE ◆ = 3–6 points ★ = 7–9 points		PRACTICE TRIAL	GRADED TRIAL #1	GRADED TRIAL #2	NOTES:
1. ★	**Perform this task out of view of patients, such as in a back office.** Verify that all petty cash expenditures have been listed on the petty cash record and that each has a receipt.				
2. ◆	Subtract all expenditures from the petty cash balance.				
3. ◆	Enter the new balance on the petty cash record.				
4. ◆	Count the money in petty cash.				
5. ◆	Verify that the petty cash amount matches the resulting amount in step 2.				
6. ◆	If the amounts do not match, verify that all subtraction was done accurately and that all receipts were entered in the petty cash record.				
7. ★	Once the account balances, obtain a check for the total expenditures from the physician or office manager.				
8. ◆	Cash the check at the bank.				
9. ◆	Enter the money in the petty cash record.				

© 2015 Pearson Education, Inc.

Name: _____

Date: _____

Document: Enter the appropriate information in the chart below. _____

Grading

Points Earned	_____		
Points Possible	_____	60	60
Percent Grade (Points Earned/Points Possible)	_____		
PASS:	_____	❏ YES ❏ NO ❏ N/A	❏ YES ❏ NO ❏ N/A

Instructor Sign-Off

Instructor: _____ **Date:** _____

© 2015 Pearson Education, Inc.

Procedure 21-7:

Reconcile a Bank Statement

Objective: Balance the clinic bank statement correctly within the time limit set by the instructor.

Supplies: Bank statement, checkbook register, calculator, blue or black pen.

Notes to the Student:

_____

_____

_____

_____

_____

_____

_____

Skills Assessment Requirements

Read and familiarize yourself with the procedure; complete the minimum practice requirements (MPRs). Document each MPR using proper charting technique. Complete each procedure within a reasonable amount of time, with a minimum of 85 percent accuracy.

© 2015 Pearson Education, Inc.

POINT VALUE ◆ = 3–6 points ★ = 7–9 points		PRACTICE TRIAL	GRADED TRIAL #1	GRADED TRIAL #2	NOTES:
1. ★	Comparing the bank statement to the checkbook register, make a check mark next to each check processed by the bank.				
2. ◆	Write the ending balance on the bank statement.				
3. ◆	Add any deposits made since the bank statement was printed.				
4. ◆	Subtract any checks not yet processed when the bank statement was printed.				
5. ◆	Add any interest awarded by the bank.				
6. ◆	Subtract any bank service fees taken by the bank.				
7. ★	If the resulting balance fails to match that in the checkbook register balance, verify that steps 1 through 6 were performed correctly.				
8. ◆	If the balances still do not match, check for addition or subtraction errors in the checkbook register.				

© 2015 Pearson Education, Inc.

Name: _____

Date: _____

Document: Enter the appropriate information in the chart below.

Grading

Points Earned	_____		
Points Possible	_____	54	54
Percent Grade (Points Earned/Points Possible)	_____		
PASS:	_____	❏ YES ❏ NO ❏ N/A	❏ YES ❏ NO ❏ N/A

Instructor Sign-Off

Instructor: _____ **Date:** _____

© 2015 Pearson Education, Inc.

Procedure 22-1:

Direct a Staff Meeting

Objective: Direct a staff meeting correctly within the time limit set by the instructor.

Supplies: Blue or black pen, paper, clock or watch to keep time, staff meeting agenda.

Affective Behaviors: Affective behaviors provide a professional approach to a skill that enhances the patient encounter. These behaviors may also display sensitivity to patients' rights, enhance communication, convey an understanding of laws and regulations, and/or provide an overall professional component to the medical assisting profession. Pay close attention to these skills, which appear in **bold, italicized** font.

Notes to the Student:

_____

_____

_____

_____

_____

_____

_____

Skills Assessment Requirements

Read and familiarize yourself with the procedure; complete the minimum practice requirements (MPRs). Document each MPR using proper charting technique. Complete each procedure within a reasonable amount of time, with a minimum of 85 percent accuracy.

© 2015 Pearson Education, Inc.

Name: _____

Date: _____

POINT VALUE ◆ = 3–6 points ★ = 7–9 points		PRACTICE TRIAL	GRADED TRIAL #1	GRADED TRIAL #2	NOTES:
1. ◆	Before the staff meeting, create an agenda of the meeting's discussion topics.				
2. ◆	**Start the meeting on time.**				
3. ◆	Note which staff are in attendance and which are absent.				
4. ◆	Discuss the agenda items one at a time, being mindful of the time.				
5. ★	**Considering time management, when non-agenda items arise, determine if they should be included in this meeting or moved to the next.**				
6. ◆	Address any issues or concerns that arise.				
7. ◆	**End the meeting at the prearranged time**.				

© 2015 Pearson Education, Inc.

Name: _____

Date: _____

Document: Enter the appropriate information in the chart below.

Grading

Points Earned	_____		
Points Possible	_____	45	45
Percent Grade (Points Earned/Points Possible)	_____		
PASS:	_____	❏ YES ❏ NO ❏ N/A	❏ YES ❏ NO ❏ N/A

Instructor Sign-Off

Instructor: _____ Date: _____

© 2015 Pearson Education, Inc.

Procedure 22-2:

Write a Job Description

Objective: Write a job description correctly within the time limit set by the instructor.

Supplies: Computer with word-processing software, list of skills needed for the position, list of duties required for the position.

Affective Behaviors: Affective behaviors provide a professional approach to a skill that enhances the patient encounter. These behaviors may also display sensitivity to patients' rights, enhance communication, convey an understanding of laws and regulations, and/or provide an overall professional component to the medical assisting profession. Pay close attention to these skills, which appear in **bold, *italicized*** font.

Notes to the Student:

_____

_____

_____

_____

_____

_____

_____

Skills Assessment Requirements

Read and familiarize yourself with the procedure; complete the minimum practice requirements (MPRs). Document each MPR using proper charting technique. Complete each procedure within a reasonable amount of time, with a minimum of 85 percent accuracy.

© 2015 Pearson Education, Inc.

Name: _____

Date: _____

POINT VALUE ◆ = 3–6 points ★ = 7–9 points		PRACTICE TRIAL	GRADED TRIAL #1	GRADED TRIAL #2	NOTES:
1. ◆	Create a title for the job position.				
2. ◆	List the name of the supervisor for the position.				
3. ★	Create a summary description of the position's duties. **Be sure that the duties fall within the scope of practice for the given job title.**				
4. ◆	List the hours required of the position.				
5. ◆	List the location of the position, when it varies.				
6. ★	**List any employment requirements (e.g., certification, malpractice insurance).**				
7. ★	**List any physical requirements for the position (e.g., lifting, prolonged sitting or standing).**				
8. ◆	Describe the evaluation process for the position.				
9. ◆	Review the job description for accuracy, as well as with the physician if needed.				

© 2015 Pearson Education, Inc.

Name: _____

Date: _____

Document: Enter the appropriate information in the chart below.

Grading

Points Earned	_____		
Points Possible	_____	63	63
Percent Grade (Points Earned/Points Possible)	_____		
PASS:	_____	❑ YES ❑ NO ❑ N/A	❑ YES ❑ NO ❑ N/A

Instructor Sign-Off

Instructor: _____ **Date:** _____

© 2015 Pearson Education, Inc.

Procedure 22-3:

Conduct an Interview

Objective: Conduct an interview correctly within the time limit set by the instructor.

Supplies: Pen, applicant's résumé.

Affective Behaviors: Affective behaviors provide a professional approach to a skill that enhances the patient encounter. These behaviors may also display sensitivity to patients' rights, enhance communication, convey an understanding of laws and regulations, and/or provide an overall professional component to the medical assisting profession. Pay close attention to these skills, which appear in **bold, *italicized*** font.

Notes to the Student:

_____
_____
_____
_____
_____
_____

Skills Assessment Requirements

Read and familiarize yourself with the procedure; complete the minimum practice requirements (MPRs). Document each MPR using proper charting technique. Complete each procedure within a reasonable amount of time, with a minimum of 85 percent accuracy.

© 2015 Pearson Education, Inc.

Name: _____

Date: _____

	POINT VALUE ◆ = 3–6 points ★ = 7–9 points	PRACTICE TRIAL	GRADED TRIAL #1	GRADED TRIAL #2	NOTES:
1. ◆	Before meeting the applicant, read the résumé.				
2. ◆	Highlight any areas of concern or interest on the résumé.				
3. ◆	Highlight résumé items that apply to the position being filled.				
4. ◆	**Greet the applicant while making direct eye contact, and state your name.**				
5. ◆	**Use a firm handshake to shake hands with the applicant.**				
6. ◆	Lead the applicant to a private room.				
7. ◆	Show the applicant where to sit for the interview.				
8. ◆	Ask the applicant about his or her potential to perform the job.				
9. ★	Review any areas of concern highlighted on the résumé.				
10. ★	Review the job description.				
11. ◆	Verify the applicant's ability to perform the required tasks.				
12. ◆	Ask the applicant if he or she has any questions about the office or physicians.				
13. ◆	Take note of any pertinent information.				
14. ◆	**Provide a decision date for the position.**				
15. ◆	**Thank the applicant, and escort the applicant out of the office.**				

© 2015 Pearson Education, Inc.

Name: _____

Date: _____

Document: Enter the appropriate information in the chart below.

Grading

Points Earned	_____		
Points Possible	_____	96	96
Percent Grade (Points Earned/Points Possible)	_____		
PASS:	_____	❏ YES ❏ NO ❏ N/A	❏ YES ❏ NO ❏ N/A

Instructor Sign-Off

Instructor: _____ **Date:** _____

© 2015 Pearson Education, Inc.

Procedure 22-4:

Call Employee References

Objective: Call for an employee reference correctly within the time limit set by the instructor.

Supplies: Telephone, employee résumé, pen.

Affective Behaviors: Affective behaviors provide a professional approach to a skill that enhances the patient encounter. These behaviors may also display sensitivity to patients' rights, enhance communication, convey an understanding of laws and regulations, and/or provide an overall professional component to the medical assisting profession. Pay close attention to these skills, which appear in **_bold, italicized_** font.

Notes to the Student:

_____

_____

_____

_____

_____

_____

Skills Assessment Requirements

Read and familiarize yourself with the procedure; complete the minimum practice requirements (MPRs). Document each MPR using proper charting technique. Complete each procedure within a reasonable amount of time, with a minimum of 85 percent accuracy.

© 2015 Pearson Education, Inc.

Name: _____

Date: _____

POINT VALUE ◆ = 3–6 points ★ = 7–9 points		PRACTICE TRIAL	GRADED TRIAL #1	GRADED TRIAL #2	NOTES:
1. ◆	Call the applicant's previous employer.				
2. ◆	Ask to speak with the office manager or supervisor.				
3. ★	*In a friendly voice, identify yourself and give the reason for the call.*				
4. ◆	Ask the previous employer open-ended questions about the employee.				
5. ◆	Ask the previous employer if the employee would be eligible for rehire.				
6. ★	Ask specifics as to the employee's job duties and job performance.				
7. ★	Ask the previous employer for any other relevant information.				
8. ◆	Note all of the previous employer's statements.				
9. ◆	*Thank the previous employer and end the phone call in a polite manner.*				

© 2015 Pearson Education, Inc.

Name: _____

Date: _____

Document: Enter the appropriate information in the chart below.

Grading

Points Earned	_____		
Points Possible	_____	63	63
Percent Grade (Points Earned/Points Possible)	_____		
PASS:	_____	❏ YES ❏ NO ❏ N/A	❏ YES ❏ NO ❏ N/A

Instructor Sign-Off

Instructor: _____ **Date:** _____

© 2015 Pearson Education, Inc.

Procedure 22-5:

Perform an Employee Evaluation

Objective: Perform an employee evaluation correctly within the time limit set by the instructor.

Supplies: Employee evaluation form, pen.

Affective Behaviors: Affective behaviors provide a professional approach to a skill that enhances the patient encounter. These behaviors may also display sensitivity to patients' rights, enhance communication, convey an understanding of laws and regulations, and/or provide an overall professional component to the medical assisting profession. Pay close attention to these skills, which appear in **bold, *italicized*** font.

Notes to the Student:

_____

_____

_____

_____

_____

_____

_____

Skills Assessment Requirements

Read and familiarize yourself with the procedure; complete the minimum practice requirements (MPRs). Document each MPR using proper charting technique. Complete each procedure within a reasonable amount of time, with a minimum of 85 percent accuracy.

© 2015 Pearson Education, Inc.

Name: _____

Date: _____

POINT VALUE ◆ = 3–6 points ★ = 7–9 points		PRACTICE TRIAL	GRADED TRIAL #1	GRADED TRIAL #2	NOTES:
1. ★	Before the evaluation meeting, ask the employee to complete a self-evaluation form on job performance. Be sure to include job performance goals for the next year.				
2. ◆	**Meet with the employee at a prearranged time and in a private room.**				
3. ◆	Compare the employee's self-evaluation form with your evaluation.				
4. ◆	Address any discrepancies between the two evaluations.				
5. ◆	**Address any areas of concern in performance or behavior while maintaining a professional manner.**				
6. ◆	Review the goals of the last evaluation and discuss progress toward those goals.				
7. ◆	Review the goals set for the next evaluation and set timelines as needed.				
8. ◆	Discuss any pay raise associated with the employee's performance.				
9. ★	Have the employee sign the employee evaluation.				
10. ◆	Place the evaluation in the employee's personnel file.				
11. ◆	**Raise any concerns about the performance evaluation with the physician.**				

© 2015 Pearson Education, Inc.

Name: _____

Date: _____

Document: Enter the appropriate information in the chart below.

Grading

Points Earned	_____		
Points Possible	_____	72	72
Percent Grade (Points Earned/Points Possible)	_____		
PASS:	_____	❑ YES ❑ NO ❑ N/A	❑ YES ❑ NO ❑ N/A

Instructor Sign-Off

Instructor: _____ **Date:** _____

© 2015 Pearson Education, Inc.

Procedure 22-6:

Discipline an Employee

Objective: Discipline an employee correctly within the time limit set by the instructor.

Supplies: Pen, paper.

Affective Behaviors: Affective behaviors provide a professional approach to a skill that enhances the patient encounter. These behaviors may also display sensitivity to patients' rights, enhance communication, convey an understanding of laws and regulations, and/or provide an overall professional component to the medical assisting profession. Pay close attention to these skills, which appear in **bold, *italicized*** font.

Notes to the Student:

_____

_____

_____

_____

_____

_____

_____

Skills Assessment Requirements

Read and familiarize yourself with the procedure; complete the minimum practice requirements (MPRs). Document each MPR using proper charting technique. Complete each procedure within a reasonable amount of time, with a minimum of 85 percent accuracy.

© 2015 Pearson Education, Inc.

POINT VALUE ◆ = 3–6 points ★ = 7–9 points		PRACTICE TRIAL	GRADED TRIAL #1	GRADED TRIAL #2	NOTES:
1. ★	*Verify all facts before meeting with the employee.*				
2. ◆	Write a disciplinary notice that contains the reason for the discipline and the action to be taken by the office and/or by the employee as a result.				
3. ◆	Request a meeting with the employee.				
4. ◆	*Hold the meeting in a private room.*				
5. ◆	Let the employee know the reason for the meeting.				
6. ◆	Discuss the disciplinary action being levied on the employee. *This should be done in a calm voice.*				
7. ◆	Discuss your expectations of the employee.				
8. ◆	Discuss the outcome if the employee's behavior does not change. *It is important not to threaten, but rather to state the facts of the situation.*				
9. ★	Ask the employee to sign the disciplinary statement.				
10. ★	If the employee refuses to sign the statement, make a note on the statement of "Contents reviewed with employee. Employee refused to sign." Affix your signature and date the document.				

© 2015 Pearson Education, Inc.

11. ◆	Place the statement in the employee's personnel record.				
12. ◆	Agree to a future date on which you will meet with the employee to discuss progress.				
13. ★	*Inform the physician of the meeting's outcome.*				

© 2015 Pearson Education, Inc.

Name: _____

Date: _____

Document: Enter the appropriate information in the chart below.

Grading

Points Earned	_____		
Points Possible	_____	90	90
Percent Grade (Points Earned/Points Possible)	_____		
PASS:	_____	❑ YES ❑ NO ❑ N/A	❑ YES ❑ NO ❑ N/A

Instructor Sign-Off

Instructor: _____ Date: _____

© 2015 Pearson Education, Inc.

Name: _____

Date: _____

Procedure 22-7:

Terminate an Employee

Objective: Terminate an employee correctly within the time limit set by the instructor.

Supplies: Pen, paper.

Affective Behaviors: Affective behaviors provide a professional approach to a skill that enhances the patient encounter. These behaviors may also display sensitivity to patients' rights, enhance communication, convey an understanding of laws and regulations, and/or provide an overall professional component to the medical assisting profession. Pay close attention to these skills, which appear in **_bold, italicized_** font.

Notes to the Student:

_____

_____

_____

_____

_____

_____

_____

Skills Assessment Requirements

Read and familiarize yourself with the procedure; complete the minimum practice requirements (MPRs). Document each MPR using proper charting technique. Complete each procedure within a reasonable amount of time, with a minimum of 85 percent accuracy.

© 2015 Pearson Education, Inc.

Name: _____

Date: _____

POINT VALUE ◆ = 3–6 points ★ = 7–9 points	PRACTICE TRIAL	GRADED TRIAL #1	GRADED TRIAL #2	NOTES:
1. ◆ **Take the employee to a private room.**				
2. ★ **In a calm and collected manner,** discuss the reason for termination.				
3. ◆ Ask the employee to return any office items, such as keys or identification badges.				
4. ◆ **Escort the employee to the workstation to collect personal belongings.**				
5. ◆ **Escort the employee from the building.**				
6. ◆ If the employee is loud or abusive, **ask the employee to leave immediately and inform the employee that personal belongings will be sent.**				
7. ★ Note the meeting's outcome in the employee's personnel file.				
8. ★ **Notify the physician of the meeting's outcome.**				

© 2015 Pearson Education, Inc.

Name: _____

Date: _____

Document: Enter the appropriate information in the chart below.

Grading

Points Earned	_____		
Points Possible	_____	57	57
Percent Grade (Points Earned/Points Possible)	_____		
PASS:	_____	❏ YES ❏ NO ❏ N/A	❏ YES ❏ NO ❏ N/A

Instructor Sign-Off

Instructor: _____ **Date:** _____

© 2015 Pearson Education, Inc.

Procedure 22-8:

File a Medical Incident Report

Objective: Fill out an incident report correctly within the time limit set by the instructor.

Supplies: Incident report form, blue or black ink pen, patient's chart.

Affective Behaviors: Affective behaviors provide a professional approach to a skill that enhances the patient encounter. These behaviors may also display sensitivity to patients' rights, enhance communication, convey an understanding of laws and regulations, and/or provide an overall professional component to the medical assisting profession. Pay close attention to these skills, which appear in **bold, italicized** font.

Notes to the Student: _____

_____

_____

_____

_____

_____

_____

_____

Skills Assessment Requirements

Read and familiarize yourself with the procedure; complete the minimum practice requirements (MPRs). Document each MPR using proper charting technique. Complete each procedure within a reasonable amount of time, with a minimum of 85 percent accuracy.

© 2015 Pearson Education, Inc.

POINT VALUE ◆ = 3–6 points ★ = 7–9 points		PRACTICE TRIAL	GRADED TRIAL #1	GRADED TRIAL #2	NOTES:
1. ★	Complete all areas of the incident report form using only facts, not opinions or judgments. For inapplicable areas, enter "NA" or "Not applicable."				
2. ★	Sign and date the form.				
3. ◆	Give the form to the office manager or office director.				
4. ◆	*Participate in any educational meetings to determine how similar events could be avoided.*				

© 2015 Pearson Education, Inc.

Name: _____

Date: _____

Document: Enter the appropriate information in the chart below.

Grading

Points Earned	_____		
Points Possible	_____	30	30
Percent Grade (Points Earned/Points Possible)	_____		
PASS:	_____	❏ YES ❏ NO ❏ N/A	❏ YES ❏ NO ❏ N/A

Instructor Sign-Off

Instructor: _____ Date: _____

© 2015 Pearson Education, Inc.

Procedure 22-9:

Use Personal Protective Equipment

Objective: Properly don and remove latex examination gloves within the time limit set by the instructor.

Supplies: Latex or non-latex gloves.

Notes to the Student:

_____

_____

_____

_____

_____

_____

Skills Assessment Requirements

Read and familiarize yourself with the procedure; complete the minimum practice requirements (MPRs). Document each MPR using proper charting technique. Complete each procedure within a reasonable amount of time, with a minimum of 85 percent accuracy.

© 2015 Pearson Education, Inc.

Name: _____

Date: _____

POINT VALUE ◆ = 3–6 points ★ = 7–9 points		PRACTICE TRIAL	GRADED TRIAL #1	GRADED TRIAL #2	NOTES:
1. ★	Wash hands.				
2. ◆	Holding the rim of the left glove with the right hand, pull on the left glove.				
3. ◆	Holding the rim of the right glove with the left hand, pull on the right glove.				
4. ◆	Smooth both gloves onto the hands.				
5. ★	If after application the glove rips or is defective, discard the glove and don a new pair. Latex gloves begin to deteriorate after 15 minutes.				
6. ◆	To remove the gloves, with the right hand pinch the center of the left glove and pull off the left glove.				
7. ◆	Hold the left glove in the right hand.				
8. ◆	With the exposed left hand, cautiously place the first two fingers of the left hand under the rim of the right glove.				
9. ◆	Push off the right glove and over the left glove, rendering the right glove inside out.				
10. ◆	Place the removed gloves in the proper disposal container.				
11. ★	Wash hands.				

© 2015 Pearson Education, Inc.

Name: _____

Date: _____

Document: Enter the appropriate information in the chart below.

Grading

Points Earned	_____		
Points Possible	_____	75	75
Percent Grade (Points Earned/Points Possible)	_____		
PASS:	_____	❏ YES ❏ NO ❏ N/A	❏ YES ❏ NO ❏ N/A

Instructor Sign-Off

Instructor: _____ Date: _____

© 2015 Pearson Education, Inc.

Procedure 22-10:

Develop an Exposure Control Plan

Objective: Develop an exposure control plan within the time limit set by the instructor.

Supplies: List of personal protective equipment within the office, training manual.

Affective Behaviors: Affective behaviors provide a professional approach to a skill that enhances the patient encounter. These behaviors may also display sensitivity to patients' rights, enhance communication, convey an understanding of laws and regulations, and/or provide an overall professional component to the medical assisting profession. Pay close attention to these skills, which appear in **bold, *italicized*** font.

Notes to the Student: _____

_____
_____
_____
_____
_____
_____

Skills Assessment Requirements _____

Read and familiarize yourself with the procedure; complete the minimum practice requirements (MPRs). Document each MPR using proper charting technique. Complete each procedure within a reasonable amount of time, with a minimum of 85 percent accuracy.

© 2015 Pearson Education, Inc.

POINT VALUE ◆ = 3–6 points ★ = 7–9 points	PRACTICE TRIAL	GRADED TRIAL #1	GRADED TRIAL #2	NOTES:
1. ◆ List each piece of personal protective equipment in the office.				
2. ◆ List the situations when each piece of equipment should/must be used.				
3. ★ **Hold an in-office training session to review each item and to discuss its use. Discuss the use in terms understood by all in the office.**				
4. ◆ Demonstrate each item's use.				
5. ◆ **Discuss how the office can reduce or eliminate exposures in the office.**				
6. ◆ **Discuss the steps the employees should take in the event of exposure.**				
7. ★ Document everything discussed at the meeting, and **distribute copies to all staff.**				

© 2015 Pearson Education, Inc.

Name: _____

Date: _____

Document: Enter the appropriate information in the chart below.

Grading

Points Earned	_____		
Points Possible	_____	48	48
Percent Grade (Points Earned/Points Possible)	_____		
PASS:	_____	❏ YES ❏ NO ❏ N/A	❏ YES ❏ NO ❏ N/A

Instructor Sign-Off

Instructor: _____ **Date:** _____

© 2015 Pearson Education, Inc.

Procedure 22-11:

Use Proper Lifting Techniques

Objective: Lift an item using the proper lifting techniques within the time limit set by the instructor.

Supplies: Item to lift.

Notes to the Student:

_____

_____

_____

_____

_____

_____

_____

Skills Assessment Requirements

Read and familiarize yourself with the procedure; complete the minimum practice requirements (MPRs). Document each MPR using proper charting technique. Complete each procedure within a reasonable amount of time, with a minimum of 85 percent accuracy.

© 2015 Pearson Education, Inc.

POINT VALUE ◆ = 3–6 points ★ = 7–9 points		PRACTICE TRIAL	GRADED TRIAL #1	GRADED TRIAL #2	NOTES:
1. ◆	Examine the item to be lifted.				
2. ★	While bending at the knees, not the waist, with feet shoulder width apart, grasp the item with both hands.				
3. ◆	Stand with the item held close to the body.				
4. ★	Place the item down, bending at the knees, not at the waist, and keeping the back straight.				

© 2015 Pearson Education, Inc.

Name: _____

Date: _____

Document: Enter the appropriate information in the chart below.

Grading

Points Earned	_____		
Points Possible	_____	30	30
Percent Grade (Points Earned/Points Possible)	_____		
PASS:	_____	❏ YES ❏ NO ❏ N/A	❏ YES ❏ NO ❏ N/A

Instructor Sign-Off

Instructor: _____ Date: _____

© 2015 Pearson Education, Inc.

Procedure 24-1:

Write an Effective Résumé

Objective: Compose your résumé correctly within the time limit set by the instructor.

Supplies: Computer with word-processing software.

Affective Behaviors: Affective behaviors provide a professional approach to a skill that enhances the patient encounter. These behaviors may also display sensitivity to patients' rights, enhance communication, convey an understanding of laws and regulations, and/or provide an overall professional component to the medical assisting profession. Pay close attention to these skills, which appear in **_bold, italicized_** font.

Notes to the Student:

_____

_____

_____

_____

_____

_____

_____

Skills Assessment Requirements

Read and familiarize yourself with the procedure; complete the minimum practice requirements (MPRs). Document each MPR using proper charting technique. Complete each procedure within a reasonable amount of time, with a minimum of 85 percent accuracy.

© 2015 Pearson Education, Inc.

Name: _____

Date: _____

POINT VALUE ♦ = 3–6 points ★ = 7–9 points	PRACTICE TRIAL	GRADED TRIAL #1	GRADED TRIAL #2	NOTES:
1. ♦ Choose a résumé template in the word-processing program.				
2. ♦ Enter your name, address, telephone number, and e-mail address.				
3. ♦ Enter an objective (e.g., "To obtain a position as a certified medical assistant in a medical practice where my skills can be used to their full potential").				
4. ♦ Enter your educational background, including degrees, in chronological order. **Never exaggerate or falsify this information.**				
5. ♦ Enter your employment history, including dates, in chronological order. **Never exaggerate or falsify this information.**				
6. ♦ List references or a phrase like, "References available upon request."				
7. ★ **Review the document for typographical and grammatical errors.**				
8. ♦ Print the résumé on quality paper.				
9. ★ **Review the résumé again for typographical and grammatical errors.**				

© 2015 Pearson Education, Inc.

Name: _____

Date: _____

Document: Enter the appropriate information in the chart below.

Grading

Points Earned	_____		
Points Possible	_____	60	60
Percent Grade (Points Earned/Points Possible)	_____		
PASS:	_____	❏ YES ❏ NO ❏ N/A	❏ YES ❏ NO ❏ N/A

Instructor Sign-Off

Instructor: _____ **Date:** _____

© 2015 Pearson Education, Inc.

Procedure 24-2:

Compose a Cover Letter

Objective: Compose a cover letter correctly within the time limit set by the instructor.

Supplies: Computer with word-processing software.

Affective Behaviors: Affective behaviors provide a professional approach to a skill that enhances the patient encounter. These behaviors may also display sensitivity to patients' rights, enhance communication, convey an understanding of laws and regulations, and/or provide an overall professional component to the medical assisting profession. Pay close attention to these skills, which appear in **bold, *italicized*** font.

Notes to the Student:

_____

_____

_____

_____

_____

_____

_____

Skills Assessment Requirements

Read and familiarize yourself with the procedure; complete the minimum practice requirements (MPRs). Document each MPR using proper charting technique. Complete each procedure within a reasonable amount of time, with a minimum of 85 percent accuracy.

© 2015 Pearson Education, Inc.

Name: _____

Date: _____

POINT VALUE ◆ = 3–6 points ★ = 7–9 points		PRACTICE TRIAL	GRADED TRIAL #1	GRADED TRIAL #2	NOTES:
1. ◆	Using the word-processing software, enter the date and name, company, and address of the letter recipient.				
2. ★	Compose a letter that addresses the desired job and the reasons the employer should consider you for the position.				
3. ◆	List any information that directly relates to your ability to perform the desired job. **Never exaggerate or be untruthful about your experience.**				
4. ★	Request an interview.				
5. ◆	State that you will call the employer to follow up in a few days.				

© 2015 Pearson Education, Inc.

Name: _____

Date: _____

Document: Enter the appropriate information in the chart below.

Grading

Points Earned	_____		
Points Possible	_____	36	36
Percent Grade (Points Earned/Points Possible)	_____		
PASS:	_____	❏ YES ❏ NO ❏ N/A	❏ YES ❏ NO ❏ N/A

Instructor Sign-Off

Instructor: _____ **Date:** _____

© 2015 Pearson Education, Inc.

Procedure 24-3:

Follow Up after an Interview

Objective: Follow up after an interview with a thank-you note to the potential employer correctly within the time limit set by the instructor.

Supplies: Note card, blue or black ink pen.

Affective Behaviors: Affective behaviors provide a professional approach to a skill that enhances the patient encounter. These behaviors may also display sensitivity to patients' rights, enhance communication, convey an understanding of laws and regulations, and/or provide an overall professional component to the medical assisting profession. Pay close attention to these skills, which appear in **_bold, italicized_** font.

Notes to the Student:

_____

_____

_____

_____

_____

_____

Skills Assessment Requirements

Read and familiarize yourself with the procedure; complete the minimum practice requirements (MPRs). Document each MPR using proper charting technique. Complete each procedure within a reasonable amount of time, with a minimum of 85 percent accuracy.

© 2015 Pearson Education, Inc.

POINT VALUE ◆ = 3–6 points ★ = 7–9 points		PRACTICE TRIAL	GRADED TRIAL #1	GRADED TRIAL #2	NOTES:
1. ◆	*Handwrite or type a note to the interviewer.*				
2. ◆	Thank the person for the interview time.				
3. ★	List something about the position or office that inspires you to want to work there.				
4. ◆	Express a desire to meet again.				
5. ★	*Send the note immediately after the interview.*				

© 2015 Pearson Education, Inc.

Name: _____

Date: _____

Document: Enter the appropriate information in the chart below.

Grading

Points Earned	_____		
Points Possible	_____	36	36
Percent Grade (Points Earned/Points Possible)	_____		
PASS:	_____	❏ YES ❏ NO ❏ N/A	❏ YES ❏ NO ❏ N/A

Instructor Sign-Off

Instructor: _____ **Date:** _____

© 2015 Pearson Education, Inc.